Medical Advances

Medical Advances

LAWRENCE GALTON

CROWN PUBLISHERS, INC./NEW YORK

Inquiries should be addressed to
Crown Publishers, Inc., One Park Avenue, New York, N.Y. 10016

Printed in the United States of America
Published simultaneously in Canada by
General Publishing Company Limited

Designed by Shari de Miskey

Library of Congress Cataloging in Publication Data

Galton, Lawrence.
  Medical advances.

  Includes bibliographical references and index.
  1. Medicine, Popular. I. Title.
DNLM: 1. Medicine—Popular works. WB130 G181n
RC82.G35 1977   615.5   77-8294
ISBN 0-517-52978-5

CONTENTS

Introduction

Many experts are wary of the dissemination of technical information. They are fearful of causing hypochondriasis; they are concerned with fostering loss of confidence in the physician; they predict aggravation of the malpractice problem; they say it may promote quackery. Such considerations must be kept in perspective. The advantages of an informed public far outweigh the possible occasional abuse or shortcomings.

Medical and health practice in the United States of America is being redefined, restructured, and refinanced. How services are to be delivered may change, but what is delivered will depend on an informed public ready to assume responsibility for its own care, knowing what information, technology, and professional skills are available. Knowledge and its use in the service of humankind is the foundation of good health and good treatment. To stay abreast of the knowledge explosion is the challenge.

But what can one do for oneself to ensure good health and good treatment? Are we not captives of fate, finances, and physicians?

Information is the key to decision and action. All of us need to know when to seek help, how to interpret the language of the diseased body, and how to communicate with health professionals. Claims and counterclaims on medical breakthroughs have become NEWS. How does one get valid and reliable interpretation of these technical matters? Surely no one—including doctors—can read all the medical journals.

Lawrence Galton has given us a way. In this book, he has abstracted a large, important, and interesting group of medical data and translated these findings into an easily readable, well-organized form. For the reader who seeks more detailed information he has included a complete reference list. It is important to note that the opinions given are those of the physicians and scientists and not those of Mr. Galton. It is even more important to note that he has not limited his review to advances against the glamour diseases of the day. He has included information on an unusually broad spectrum of conditions. This is health education that is credible.

—Theodore Cooper, M.D.
Dean, Cornell University
Medical College

CHAPTER 1

About—and How to Use— This Book

This book is NOT a general treatise on medicine and health. It bears no relationship to any home medical adviser or encyclopedia.

Rather, its aim is to alert you to the newest specific developments in medicine that you can use—or that your physician may be able to use now—to help with problems more effectively, more simply, more safely, or more inexpensively than in the past, and even to solve some problems that may have been unyielding before.

Many of these advances result from extended large-scale trials with hundreds and thousands of patients by many investigators at many major clinical and research centers throughout the world.

But there are other advances as well—new insights and treatment methods arrived at by individual physicians (sometimes because they personally were sufferers, sometimes because they were alert enough to pick up valuable clues from accidental events and even the experiences of observant patients). And while many of these are not necessarily of earthshaking importance on the total scientific scene, they nevertheless can be of possibly great importance to individuals with annoying, even if not life-threatening, disturbances.

The range is broad:

• From a simple treatment for hay fever worked out by one physician for himself after no usual treatment helped for twenty years, a treatment which he has, modestly, suggested may possibly be helpful to others (it has been) . . . to markedly improved regimens for controlling and sometimes curing the life-threatening diseases: cancers (breast, bone, lung, and others), heart diseases, kidney diseases, and more.

• From new insights into chronic heartburn and its treatment to eating patterns as therapy (and even prophylaxis) for many other gastrointestinal problems . . . to new methods of managing disturbances of vision, hearing, taste, and smell.

• What's new for headaches includes a remarkable medication previously used for heart trouble and now used for migraine . . . and the use of novel methods for cluster, tension, muscle spasm, and other types of headache.

• There are new developments for pain, palsy, pregnancy, and a striking advance for Paget's bone disease, which affects two and a half million Americans, many of them unaware of being affected.

• There are also new insights and treatments for respiratory problems, including asthma and the common cold—and many for skin disorders ranging from acne and psoriasis to extreme light sensitivity.

• The breadth of helpful new knowledge is great, extending even to the problem of "airplane ankle," to the misuse of the bed by insomniacs and a good way to learn to fall asleep if you're one of them, and to hangovers, nightmares, sleepwalking, and stuttering, and what can now be done for them.

• All told, you will find more than three hundred entries, which can be found either under the general chapter headings or by turning to the Index and looking under the specific symptom or problem.

Although there are some developments you may apply on your own, this is not a self-treatment book. It is, however, intended very much to provide self-help—in the sense that you may be encouraged by a new development to seek help where you haven't before, or, again, because help was inadequate.

Because physicians are busy and the medical literature on new developments is so vast that it is difficult for them to keep up with everything (even in their own specialized fields), it would be understandable if your physician was not aware of a new development that could hold promise for you.

If you inform him, he could check further.

To help you both, each entry here carries a reference to a list (see the References section at the end of the book) showing the physician or physicians who reported the development or the medical journal or other source that supplied the report.

CHAPTER 2

Allergies

Not including the more than eight million with asthma (see Respiratory Diseases), which is commonly allergic in nature but may involve other factors, some twenty-two million Americans have allergy problems.

About thirteen and a half million have the nonasthmatic type of rhinitis, or inflammation of the nasal passages, often called hay fever when it is seasonal and perennial when it occurs year round. More than eight and a half million have other types of allergies, including skin allergies, particularly hives and some types of eczema, and hypersensitivity to foods, drugs, and insect stings.

These are recent developments that may be helpful to allergy sufferers:

A new protection schedule for the insect-sensitive

Hypersensitivity to the stings of bees, wasps, and other insects can produce severe local reactions with swellings of unusual size and duration or general reactions with hives and overall itching. Super-sensitivity can also lead to anaphylactic shock, a combination of signs and symptoms including generalized swelling, chest tightness, ab-dominal pain, nausea, dizziness, speech difficulties, weakness, rapid blood-pressure fall, and unconsciousness. Each year, anaphylactic shock from insect stings kills some fifty people in the United States.

For some years, protection for the hypersensitive has been possible with hyposensitization, achieved through a series of injections of first small, then gradually increasing doses of insect extracts to build up resistance, followed by regular maintenance injections at frequent intervals throughout the year.

Now a much simpler schedule of maintenance injections will be welcome news, thanks to a ten-year study of 397 insect-sensitive patients by physicians of the American Academy of Allergy Commit-tee on Insects. Patients receiving maintenance injections at intervals of every two to three months have been found to do as well as those receiving them every four weeks, saving on visits to physicians and on costs. The mechanics of why this is so are not entirely clear, but obviously the patients are getting the same level of protection. (A-1)

"Confessions of a physician with hay fever—with a short note on what to do about it"

Hay fever is no serious threat to life but as any victim knows it can seriously interfere with work and pleasure. Ragweed pollen is the major offender, but other wind-pollenated weeds, grasses, and trees can bring on attacks. Victims spend hundreds of millions yearly for antihistamines, anticongestants, and other medications, and for injec-tions aimed at hyposensitization.

Is there some simple, effective, not generally used way to lick hay fever?

For the first time, in 1973, a physician's newspaper, *Medical Tribune*, published a little essay called "Confessions of a Physician With Hay Fever—With a Short Note on What to Do about It." The physician is the distinguished Donald J. Dalessio, head of the Division of Neurology, Scripps Clinic and Research Foundation, LaJolla, California. Each year for twenty years he suffered from hay fever, the symptoms beginning in late April, raging through May, June, and July, and beginning to taper in August.

He had surveyed all the usual treatments and was far from impressed with any of them. He disliked consuming quantities of medicine, including antihistamines, which dulled him, and anticongestants, which made him anxious.

Finally, he arrived at his own method of treatment. On awakening each morning during his hay fever season, he applies a small amount of a potent corticosteroid (cortisonelike) cream with his fifth finger to the nasal mucous membranes, using either flumethasone, 0.03%, or fluocinonide, 0.05%. Only a small amount is necessary, he emphasizes. The cream causes slight nasal irritation, and he often snuffs vigorously, inhaling the cream to the upper reaches of the mucous membranes in the nose. At night, the process is repeated, and before going to bed he takes a 6-milligram dose of Polaramine, which provides antihistamine effects (at night pollen counts rise and the drug's sedative reaction is hardly bothersome).

Allergy was not Dr. Dalessio's field and he hadn't made any studies (medical men, before using any new treatment, usually like to have large-scale studies with many patients under scientifically controlled conditions). "I can only say," he wrote, "that if it works for me, it may work for you." An occasional sneeze still occurs, a little tickling may appear during the day, but nasal discharge is much reduced and paroxysmal sneezing is almost eliminated.

That was in 1973. Not long ago, the medical newspaper reprinted Dr. Dalessio's essay at the request of a Philadelphia physician, Dr. Peter B. Bloom, so that others could benefit from it.

Since his internship thirteen years ago, Dr. Bloom had told his colleagues he would award them a thousand dollars on the spot if they would cure him of his August-October hay fever. He'd had it since he was five and had continued to have it despite desensitization, antihistamines, and constant air conditioning. And having finished his training in both internal medicine and psychiatry, he had found no evidence that his hay fever was psychosomatic.

However, he points out, "since taking Dr. Dalessio's advice—even modifying it to applying fluocinonide 0.05% every two-three days and without Polaramine, I have been completely free of any symptoms whatsoever. Only fellow hay fever sufferers will understand the true significance of having dry handkerchiefs from August to October.

"Dr. Dalessio and I have exchanged letters and while I have sobered regarding the $1,000, I've already sent him an equivalent amount of my appreciation."   (A-2)

(The preparations are available only on prescription, but an open-minded physician may be willing to prescribe them for you for a trial.)

Easing year-round allergic rhinitis

Home humidification during the winter often can be surprisingly helpful for people with perennial or year-round allergic rhinitis. So a study with 817 patients indicates.

Carried on for three winters, the study found that with humidification previous winter-long symptoms of dryness in the nose, throat, and deep chest were markedly reduced; breathing improved and permitted more restful sleep; the need to clear the breathing passages of mucus in the morning lessened. In addition, 83 percent of the patients were free of respiratory infections during the winters for the first time in years. In homes with hot air systems, humidification can be achieved by a device that attaches to the system or furnace; in other homes or apartments this can be done through room humidifiers.   (A-3)

Mold allergy and nasal congestion

Sensitivity to molds can, in itself, sometimes produce nasal congestion, stuffiness, and other annoying symptoms. The sensitivity also tends to occur along with other sensitivities such as pollen allergy.

That many patients can be helped by learning how to avoid molds has been shown by an Indianapolis study.

Among the measures that can be used: keeping dust accumulation to a minimum and, unhappily for plant lovers, eliminating plants from the home. Both measures markedly reduce exposure to molds.

Also helpful: a dry, well-ventilated, well-lighted basement, which tends to discourage growth of molds.

A particularly effective measure—if it is possible for the family to be away from home for two or three days—is to place a coffee can containing a small amount of formaldehyde in each room of the house. Left in place for just twenty-four hours, the formaldehyde often will eliminate household molds for as long as six months. An important precaution: after use of formaldehyde, the house should be well aired.   (A-4)

Skin allergies: the prime causes identified

Although almost any substance coming in contact with the skin can, in those who happen to be sensitive to it, cause trouble—redness, rash, and itching—a study carried out by Dr. E. J. Rudner of Detroit and teams of dermatologists at ten major medical centers now has identified what are, by far, the leading troublemakers.

At the head of the list: nickel sulfate. It's often used in the making of inexpensive watches, earrings, rings, and bracelets. And as many as 11 percent of those who wear such jewelry, it turns out, eventually suffer allergic reactions.

Another major item: potassium dichromate, a substance commonly found in tanned leather. About 8 percent of the population is allergic to it.

Antiseptics, a common group of household products, are also responsible for many allergy cases. One ingredient, thimerosal, can trigger attacks in almost 10 percent of users; another, merthiolate, produces reactions in 8 percent.

And an ingredient in many hair dyes, p-phenylenediamine, produces itching and other allergy symptoms in 8 percent of users.

The purpose of the study was to let physicians in on substances most likely to be responsible for otherwise often mysterious skin problems in patients. But the results can also provide guidance for many of the victims.

The answer to such skin problems is to suspect possible culprits, track down the actual one, and remove it from contact with the skin. In many cases the patient can do this for himself.   (A-5)

The poison-ivy sensitive and cashew nuts

They were a series of patients known to be sensitive to poison ivy, poison oak, or poison sumac. But when they developed a generalized eczema outbreak, they had not been exposed to any of the poison plants.

Finally, physicians at the Hitchcock Clinic in Hanover, New Hampshire, puzzled out the problem. In each case, there had been some gobbling of raw cashew nuts (often sold now in organic food stores).

Anyone sensitive to the poison plants may do well to avoid eating cashews raw. When roasted, the nuts may produce no reaction, but in the raw state they contain sizeable amounts of shell oil on their surfaces, and the oil is much like the oleoresin of the poison plants in allergy-causing activity.   (A-6)

Apparel allergies

Mysterious itching and rash can stem from the formaldehyde used in crease-resistant fabrics. Because sensitivity to the chemical is an increasing problem, one study has looked into formaldehyde content of 112 women's fabrics.

The findings: 100 percent rayon, 100 percent cotton, 65 percent dacron-35 percent cotton, and 50 percent polyester-50 percent cotton have the highest concentration of free formaldehyde that may bother those allergic to it. Fabrics with the least amount: 100 percent polyester knit and 100 percent orlon acrylic. (A-7)

The solution to another apparel allergy mystery has been turned up in a study at the Medical College of Virginia, in Richmond. It has been known that rashes from the rubber elastic in undergarments can occur in the sensitive. But in a series of patients afflicted with what could theoretically have been rashes from such sensitivity, tests showed no allergy to the elastic itself. The trouble proved to be a laundry bleach used in washing the underwear. The bleach action on the elastic produced a chemical change that led to sensitivity. The solution to the problem is simple enough, report the investigators: use of underwear without elastic or rinsing without bleach. (A-8)

Allergic cough in children

When a child develops a barking, nonproductive cough and no obvious physical cause can be found, there is often a tendency for a physician as well as parents to consider it psychogenic or "nervous" in nature. But, at least in some cases, allergy may be responsible.

An exemplary case reported to a meeting of the American Academy of Pediatrics: a ten-year-old girl who coughed as often as every fifteen to thirty seconds. Efforts to help her had included various medications and even tonsil and adenoid removal. Her coughing, which finally led to her exclusion from school because of the disturbance it produced in the classroom, became worse whenever she was excited or tense; it then seemed especially likely to be psychogenic.

However, when allergy tests were performed, they indicated sensitivity to trees, molds, and house dust. Allergy treatment, including injections in small doses of the offending substances, eliminated the cough. There has been no recurrence over a four-year period. (A-9)

Tobacco smoke allergy on top of other allergy

About one-sixth of people allergic to pollens or other substances may also be hypersensitive to tobacco smoke, according to a study at the University of Tennessee Allergy Clinics in Memphis. There, when two hundred allergy patients were picked at random for tests of smoke sensitivity, the tests were positive in thirty-two, or 16 percent.

The sensitivity seems to occur largely in (1) women who do not themselves smoke but are exposed to tobacco smoke at home or at work, and (2) teen-agers exposed at school and in other situations when friends smoke.

The use of tolerance-building injections of tobacco extract, tried at the clinics, led to excellent relief of eye, nose, and bronchial symptoms in most cases, and to fair to good relief in the remainder.   (A-10)

The aspirin-sensitive

As valuable as it is, aspirin is not well tolerated by about 0.9 percent of the general population. But if you have other allergy problems, your chances of being allergic to aspirin are increased.

In a recent study by Dr. G. I. Settipane and other Providence, Rhode Island, physicians, 1.4 percent of people with rhinitis or nasal congestion problems for other reasons proved to be sensitive to aspirin. The sensitivity rate was far higher—3.8 percent—among asthmatics.

Curiously, in asthmatics the predominant manifestation of aspirin sensitivity is bronchial spasm, such as occurs in an asthma attack; in rhinitis sufferers, however, it is hives; in the general population, among those not otherwise allergic, the symptoms of aspirin intolerance are about equally divided between bronchial spasm and hives.
                                                      (A-11)

A little-known allergy: cold urticaria

Typically, the victims break out with hives—not because of allergy to a food or inhalant or chemical, but because of hypersensitivity to cold. Lips may swell and hives appear when ice cream is eaten; hands may puff up and generalized hives appear when a cold object is gripped; hives may appear and consciousness may even be lost while swimming in cold water.

Any help for such cold urticaria? Investigators at the National Jewish Hospital and Research Center, Denver, report good results in a series of patients treated with an antihistamine drug, cyproheptadine. Any physician can prescribe it for trial.   (A-12)

Food allergies: the ten most common offenders and what they trigger

By far the chief offenders among food allergens are cow's milk, chocolate and cola (the kola nut family), corn, eggs, the pea family (chiefly peanut, which is not a nut), citrus fruits, tomato, wheat and other small grains, cinnamon, and artificial food colors.

Food allergy can lead to a remarkable variety of symptoms and combinations of symptoms—so indicates a recent special report to physicians by Dr. Frederic Speer of the Speer Allergy Clinic, Shawnee Mission, Kansas, in *American Family Physician*, a medical journal.

Cow's milk is the most common food allergen—just as important among adults as children. Among its most frequent manifestations: constipation, diarrhea, constipation alternating with diarrhea, distension, nonlocalized abdominal pain; also, nasal and bronchial congestion, with excessive production of mucus.

Chocolate and cola, from the same kola nut family, often produce the same problems, headache being the most common. The two substances in some cases are important factors in asthma, perennial rhinitis, and eczema.

Corn sensitivity not only may produce headache, including migraine. It can lead to allergic tension (insomnia, irritability, restlessness, oversensitivity) and allergic fatigue (sleepiness, torpor, weakness, vague aching).

Egg may cause almost any allergic manifestation, and is most likely to cause hives and angioedema (also called giant hives and characterized by the sudden temporary appearance of large skin and mucous membrane wheals and intense itching). Egg also may be involved in eczema, asthma, headache, and gastrointestinal allergy.

In the pea family, the most common offender is the peanut. Mature beans and peas are more often problems than are green peas and snap beans. Pea family members can commonly cause headache and may be factors in asthma, hives, and angioedema.

Oranges, lemons, limes, grapefruits, and tangerines can induce eczema and hives and are sometimes factors in canker sores (aphthous stomatitis) and asthma.

Tomato is a common cause of eczema, hives, and canker sores. It seldom induces headache but may cause asthma.

The small grains include wheat, rice, barley, oats, wild rice, millet, and rye. Wheat is the most allergenic, rye, the least. Rye often can be used as a substitute when wheat is the problem. Manifestations of grain allergy include asthma and gastrointestinal disturbances.

Cinnamon is a leading cause of hives and headache, and an occasional cause of asthma.

Artificial food colors are used in carbonated beverages, breakfast drinks, bubble gum, gelatin desserts, and many medications. The most important allergens among them are the red dye amaranth and the yellow dye tartrazine. Common symptoms of food color allergy are hives and asthma.

Other food allergens include pork, beef, onion, garlic, white potato, fish of all kinds, coffee, shrimp, banana, walnut, and pecan. Almost any other food may be allergenic for some people.

Foods least likely to be troublesome: chicken, turkey, lamb, rabbit; beet, spinach, cabbage, cauliflower, broccoli, turnip, Brussels sprouts, squash, lettuce, carrot, celery, sweet potato; plum, cherry, apricot, cranberry, blueberry, fig; tea, olives, tapioca, sugar.

This is the advice the report has to offer physicians about management of food allergy:

The first step should be differential diagnosis, which means a check to make certain that something serious other than allergy is not involved.

Next, a history, which may provide clues from when a patient's attacks occur and what foods may have been eaten prior to them.

If one food is suspected, it is removed from the diet for three weeks. If symptoms subside, the food is then reintroduced to see if it returns the symptoms. If several foods are suspected, all are removed from the diet for three weeks. One is then returned to the diet and later, at intervals of two days, the others are returned to determine which one or several may be the troublemakers.   (A-13)

CHAPTER 3

Arthritis and Musculoskeletal Disorders

Arthritis: no cure, but some progress

Our most widespread chronic disorder, arthritis afflicts some twenty million Americans, about one in every eleven. Its causes remain obscure—and there is no cure.

There are many degrees of osteoarthritis (which tends to develop with advancing age and is also known by such names as "wear and tear" and "degenerative" arthritis) and of rheumatoid arthritis (a more severe, often more crippling disorder that tends to affect more women than men).

In some cases, relatively simple measures, such as use of aspirin or aspirinlike compounds, are helpful. In others, relief may be offered by a much broader program of treatment, varying with each patient, including some or all of medication, rest, exercise, physical therapy, heat, and special mechanical aids.

But there are those with more severe degrees of osteoarthritis or rheumatoid arthritis who do not benefit adequately from medical care and suffer extreme pain and crippling. Today, for many of the latter, the rapid development of joint replacement surgery offers great and growing promise.

A new drug for the arthritic

With action similar to aspirin but, in many cases, producing fewer undesirable effects when used for arthritis, Motrin is a newer compound that has become available in the United States after some years of use in Britain and Canada.

But first, let us look at aspirin, which is a remarkable drug. Along with pain- and fever-relieving activity, it is also antiinflammatory. And inflammation as well as pain is a major problem in arthritis.

Provided it is properly used, aspirin can do much for a large proportion of rheumatoid arthritics. Too often it is not properly used, perhaps because of the failure of some physicians to provide understanding for patients. As a recent American Medical Association report emphasizes, for aspirin to have antiinflammatory activity, a certain blood level—18 to 25 milligram percent—is needed. For this to be attained, 3 to 6 grams of aspirin per day (that is, 12 to 20 5-grain aspirin tablets) are required. Doses below this amount have analgesic, or pain-relieving, but little antiinflammatory effect.

Adult patients, the report indicates, usually can be started on twelve aspirin tablets daily—three taken halfway through each meal, and, again, at bedtime with food. If necessary, the dose can be gradually increased every three to five days until side effects occur. Tinnitus, or ringing in the ear, is a side effect that indicates high therapeutic blood levels of aspirin. If this occurs, the dosage is reduced by one tablet every two to three days until the tinnitus stops. If gastric upset occurs, antacids can be used liberally. And once the proper dosage is established, it can be continued for years.

In some patients, however, therapeutic dose levels of aspirin, even with antacids, produce side effects that are difficult to tolerate. For them, Motrin may be of value.

After studies abroad, trials with it in more than eight hundred patients at Emory, Northwestern, and other university medical centers indicate that the compound relieves pain, decreases morning stiffness, and improves joint motion in many patients with rheumatoid arthritis, and that it is beneficial in most people with osteoarthritis. At the same time, comparing Motrin with aspirin, such undesirable effects as nausea, heartburn, indigestion, abdominal cramps, constipation, and diarrhea are half or even less frequent with Motrin.   (AM-1)

Other drug treatments for arthritis

An often-useful additional aid along with aspirin therapy is the injection of steroids (cortisonelike compounds) into actively inflamed joints—knees, shoulders, ankles, elbows, wrists, fingers. A number of long-acting forms of such compounds—prednisone, prednisolone, triamcinolone and dexamethasone—are available and effective. The dose ranges from 2 to 12 milligrams for small joints to 20 to 40 mg. for larger ones. The effect usually lasts one to two weeks but sometimes may persist for several months. Injections may be repeated every two to three weeks for several times, then every six to eight weeks.

When patients with rheumatoid arthritis fail to respond to aspirin, more potent antimalarial drugs may be added. Hydroxychloroquine sulfate, used in doses of 200 milligrams twice a day, is effective in about 60 percent of patients. Rarely does improvement occur before six weeks and in some cases may require up to six months of treatment. Reductions of pain, stiffness, and swelling are often slowly progressive. Various side effects may occur—rash, nausea, vomiting, cramps, or diarrhea. If they occur when the drug is first begun, a lower dosage usually eliminates them. Another side effect, blurred vision, also may be eliminated by reduced dosage. Other side effects are muscle weakness and hair loss, both of which are reversible with lowered dosage or discontinuation of the drug.

Gold therapy is often helpful for rheumatoid arthritis. About 70 percent of patients able to take it improve, often with complete elimination of symptoms.

Two forms of gold in common use are gold sodium thiomalate and aurothioglucose. Gold is given weekly by intramuscular injection. Test doses—10 milligrams the first week, 25 milligrams the second and third weeks—are used to check for allergy or sensitivity to gold. Thereafter, full doses of 50 milligrams are used weekly for up to about twenty weeks.

Beneficial effects of gold usually do not appear until 500 to 800 milligrams—and, occasionally, 1,200 to 1,500—have been used. Once improvement occurs, injection frequency is decreased and then a regular maintenance program of an injection every three to five weeks is established.

The most common side effects of gold are mouth ulcers and itching skin rash, which are reversible with discontinuation of treatment, but treatment may be started again after they have cleared completely. Routine blood counts are needed to make certain that anemia or other disturbances do not develop.   (AM-2)

Blocking arthritic shooting pains

Patients who develop shooting abdominal or leg pain because of osteoarthritis or rheumatoid arthritis may now be helped by a new method of placing a combination of local anesthetic and cortisone in the low back.

The medications are injected near but outside the spinal cord at a point where certain key nerves exit from the spine. The injections, given in a series, block pain impulses and at the same time help decrease irritation of the nerves by the arthritic process.

Developed at the University of Virginia Medical School, Charlottesville, by Dr. Harold Carron, the technique has been reported to produce considerable relief and the relief appears to be presistent.

(AM-3)

Help for psoriatic arthritis

Psoriasis, a troublesome enough skin disease in itself, sometimes produces arthritic manifestations similar to those of rheumatoid arthritis. Active joint disease and pain tend to occur whenever there is a flare-up of scaly psoriasis of the skin or nails and, if uncontrolled, the arthritis can be as crippling as rheumatoid arthritis.

Now a recent study by Dr. J. Baum and other Dallas physicians indicates that 6-mercaptopurine, a compound sometimes used for leukemia, may be valuable in severe cases of psoriatic arthritis. Of a group of patients for whom it was tried, 84 percent showed improvement in both psoriasis and arthritis, usually within a period of three weeks. Improvement could be maintained with small daily doses. When treatment was stopped in one patient, the improvement continued for ten months.   (AM-4)

Treating ankylosing spondylitis

Ankylosing spondylitis is a type of arthritis that affects the small joints of the spine. There is stiffening of the spinal joints and ligaments so that movement may become increasingly painful and difficult. The stiffening may extend to the ribs, limiting the flexibility of the rib cage, so that breathing is impaired.

The disease most often affects young adults. It used to be thought to be about ten times as common in men as in women, but recent studies suggest that it may affect women fully as often as men; all told, it afflicts some three million Americans. In women, it may sometimes be thought to be rheumatoid arthritis. And some women may think their nagging back pain symptoms are due to menstrual cramps.

Ankylosing spondylitis is chronic. But if pain can be relieved so as to allow posture-maintaining exercises to be performed, it is often possible to avoid crippling and to achieve a fully productive life.

Cortisonelike drugs have not been particularly effective for ankylosing spondylitis; gold therapy has been ineffective.

However, two drugs have been found effective: phenylbutazone and indomethacin. About 90 percent of patients are satisfactorily helped by either drug. The drugs may sometimes produce side effects, which can be reversed when they are withdrawn.

But aspirin, too, may be effective in some cases. So indicates a study by a nationwide team of Veterans Administration and university hospitals investigators.

In the study, patients received aspirin for six weeks, phenylbutazone for six weeks, and indomethacin for six weeks. The medications were placed in look-alike capsules so that neither physicians nor patients knew when which drug was being used until the trial was over.

Although phenylbutazone and indomethacin proved to be superior for most patients, in 12 percent both pain relief and improvement in spinal mobility were greater with aspirin. Aspirin, the study suggests, should be given a trial for ankylosing spondylitis before resorting to other more potent and more expensive drugs.   (AM-5)

Good news for arthritics with Felty's syndrome

Of all patients with rheumatoid arthritis, 1 to 2 percent also suffer from Felty's syndrome; along with arthritis symptoms, they have an abnormally low white blood count and an enlarged spleen.

In the past, patients with this severe form of disease rarely lived more than a few years. Many died of infections because their severely depleted white blood cells could not fight off common disease-causing organisms. Removal of the enlarged spleen, suspected of destroying the white cells, helped somewhat, but for a third of the patients the reprieve was short.

Then, recently, at the Arthritis Clinical Research Center of the University of Colorado, Denver, Dr. R. C. Gupta happened to read a medical report on lithium carbonate and its use in the treatment of patients with manic-depressive illness. That psychiatric problem has nothing to do with arthritis. But, Gupta considered, a side effect of lithium carbonate—a marked increase of white blood cells—might be of some use.

On a hunch, Gupta used lithium carbonate for a patient dying of infection associated with Felty's syndrome. The patient's life was saved.

Since then, lithium carbonate has been used for six weeks at a time in a group of patients suffering from Felty's syndrome and rheumatoid arthritis. Results: most encouraging, thus far. Only time will tell whether the drug will have long-term beneficial effects and eliminate the need for spleen removal in the treatment of the disease. (AM-6)

Glove treatment for arthritic hands

A few years ago, Dr. George E. Ehrlich, director of the Arthritis Clinic at Albert Einstein Medical Center, Philadelphia, noted that several of his women patients with hands affected by rheumatoid arthritis or osteoarthritis wore stretch gloves and, when queried, reported that they helped so much that they kept them on during the night.

Intrigued, Ehrlich set up a trial with forty-four women, aged thirty-two to eighty-two, with painful hand arthritis. In all but three of the forty-four, it turned out, the stretch gloves greatly reduced or eliminated morning pain, stiffness, and joint swellings, and increased grip strength. Benefits occurred usually within the first two days of wearing the gloves, and some women reported being able to sleep through the night for the first time in many years.

Both nylon-knit and Spandex-and-nylon gloves were used and proved effective, but many patients found the latter more comfortable. The mechanism of action of the gloves is not known. A possibility suggested by Ehrlich: They may have a massaging action that helps to prevent blood pooling in the hands.   (AM-7)

Arthritis surgery and joint replacement

No area of arthritis research has progressed so far and so fast in recent years as arthritis surgery, including replacement of diseased joints with man-made prostheses.

Synovectomy. The synovium is a membrane lining body joints and producing a fluid that lubricates the joint surfaces. In severe rheumatoid arthritis, swelling and inflammation of the synovium may distend a joint, stretching and damaging ligaments and tendons, leading to deformity.

In synovectomy, swollen membrane is removed, stretched ligaments are repaired, and displaced tendons restored to normal location. The operation can be used for hands, fingers, knees, shoulders, elbows, and other joints.

Synovectomy is palliative, not curative. It appears that not all synovial membrane can be removed from a joint and there may be recurrence of disease. But in carefully selected patients the procedure may be of value.   (AM-8)

Arthrodesis. Arthrodesis is the surgical fusion of a joint. It may be used when arthritis twists and gnarls a joint, producing disabling pain and deformity. It is often effective in relieving pain and may improve function.

Fusion to fix the wrist, for example, in a neutral undeformed position has produced reportedly gratifying results in as many as 96 percent of patients, leading to increased grasping power and making the wrist pain-free and more useful. With a bone graft, the wrist is fused so that it no longer bends, but patients report that the increased function stemming from relief of pain and increased strength more than compensate for loss of bending.   (AM-9)

Hip replacement. A first dramatic prosthetic joint development about a decade ago was the artificial hip. It represented a monumental feat.

The hip, the largest joint in the body, is a ball and socket joint. It is frequently affected by both rheumatoid arthritis and osteoarthritis. With disease, the ball of the bone at the head of the thighbone, or femur, can rub against the roughened socket surface in the hip and produce intense pain.

The difficulty in replacing the joint hinged on finding a material strong enough to withstand the loads of body weight; an individual will put many millions of loading pounds on the hip in the course of ten years. The material had to be elastic enough to mimic the energy-absorbing qualities of living bone and cartilage, durable enough to last a lifetime, compatible with and uncorroded by body fluids and tissues, self-lubricating, and slip-proof.

The hip prosthesis developed by Dr. John Charnley in Reddington, England, fulfilled the criteria. It uses stainless steel or Vitallium for one component and the plastic called polyethylene for the other, with both components cemented into place.

Commonly, patients report that pain disappears immediately, even upon awakening from the anesthesia. For four or five days, the operated leg may be rested with traction in a light splint. Thereafter, patients may begin to walk with the aid of a walker, later crutches, and still later without aid.

At first, hip replacement was confined to patients sixty years of age or older because of uncertainty about how long the prosthesis might last. Now, after a decade of satisfactory experience, surgeons are implanting artificial hips in much younger patients and even in some severely afflicted children. It is estimated that, currently, as many as forty thousand people a year in this country are receiving artificial hips.   (AM-10)

Knee replacement. The knee, which bears virtually all the body's weight, is very susceptible to arthritis and is one of the most frequently affected joints.

A complex joint, it bends, rotates, locks when fully extended, and redistributes body weight during flexion and extension (without which we couldn't get up from a squatting position).

Knees sometimes have been fused to stop motion and pain. Partial prostheses including metal disks to separate the head of the thighbone and shinbone (tibia) have been used.

Although long considered an almost impossible joint to replace completely, there are now several prosthetic joints that have been used successfully in hundreds of patients. They include a "polycentric" knee, a "geometric" knee, a Freeman-Swanson knee (named for its English developers), and a UCI knee (University of California at Irvine). They differ in technical detail.

Length of rehabilitation varies from one patient to another. Some use crutches for several months; some use a walker until they feel comfortable with a cane. Some studies, such as one at Mayo Clinic, have shown that knee replacement relieves pain in 84 percent of patients, provides normal stability in 93 percent, and 78 percent need no help in walking.   (AM-11, 12)

Ankle joints. The ankle, an intricate hinge, must support entire body weight and allow the foot to tilt and rotate through many angles. Early ankle replacements were of limited use, consisting of a hinge allowing only up and down movement.

A new ankle joint, developed by Dr. Theodore Waugh at the University of California at Irvine, appears to be far superior. Consisting

of a T-shaped metal piece that screws up into the shin and a rounded
runner covering the talus ankle bone, it can be implanted in less than
an hour and provides side-to-side as well as up-and-down foot motion. Most patients are up and walking on crutches less than a week
after implantation and walking unaided within a month.

Some of the first patients to receive the new ankle joints, previously
unable for years to walk without crutches, reportedly are playing
golf.   (AM-13)

Toe implants. In some cases of severe arthritis, the foot becomes
deformed to the point that, for pain relief, one of the joints of the great
toe must be surgically removed. But the toe then loses function and
begins to drift to the side, producing new deformity and difficulty in
walking. To help in such cases, a variety of prosthetic implants,
including half-joints, spacers, and hinged devices, have been developed.

At University of California, Los Angeles, Medical Center, of the
first nineteen patients receiving twenty-five implants—the majority
middle-aged and elderly women—most have experienced pain relief
and improved toe alignment. Ten have become able to walk without
limitation, and five others are able to walk for up to six blocks at a
time, reports Dr. Andrea Cracchiolo III.   (AM-14)

Finger joints. When arthritis produces severe hand deformities—
some so grotesque that they bear such descriptive names as "Swan
neck" and "Boutonniere" (French for buttonhole)—synthetic finger
joints are often of value.

A typical finger joint implant is made of silicone rubber and can be
likened to a piece of taffy pulled out at both ends. The ends, following
removal of a deformed joint, are positioned in channels in bones, and
the center, thick part of the device lies between and keeps the bones
properly aligned.

Many thousands of the joints have been implanted in patients at
many medical centers, and the prostheses, reports Dr. Alfred B.
Swanson, a hand surgeon at Blodgett Memorial Hospital, Grand
Rapids, Michigan, who developed them, provide as much as 75 percent of the efficiency of healthy, natural joints.   (AM-15)

Knuckles. Very recently, prosthetic knuckles have been developed to help patients with arthritis-deformed hands no longer able to
grip and pinch or to open widely enough to grasp large objects.

Developed at the Hospital of the Albert Einstein College of
Medicine, Bronx, New York, by Dr. Robert J. Schultz, director of

orthopedic surgery, the knuckles are made of stainless steel and polyethylene. They can be implanted in about two hours. Patients usually begin to use their hands on the fourth day after surgery.

Although the knuckles are not perfect, they are "close," Dr. Schultz reports. Follow-up on the first one hundred fifty cases for as long as two and a half years shows no adverse reactions.   (AM-16)

Shoulder joints. Now beginning to come into use is a new shoulder joint developed by Dr. Melvin Post and other orthopedists at the Michael Reese Hospital and Medical Center, Chicago.

The joint is somewhat like the Charnley artificial hip in replacing damaged shoulder surfaces with a metal-to-plastic ball-and-socket joint. Additionally, a special plastic collar for the device locks around and helps prevent shoulder dislocation.

After the joint is implanted, the arm is immobilized for four weeks. Gentle motion exercises then are begun. Thus far, in the first few patients to receive it, the shoulder prosthesis is providing pain-free ability to carry out movements and tasks previously painful or impossible.   (AM-17)

Elbows. Many less than satisfactory artificial elbows have been developed. Failings have included limited range of motion, loosening, and need for reoperation in a significant percentage of patients.

A new joint developed at the Harvard Medical School and Robert B. Brigham Hospital, Boston, by Dr. Frederick C. Ewald has been proving much more effective in its first uses.

It consists of a cuplike plastic element and a metal component shaped somewhat like a ladle. The cup is fastened to the top of the ulna bone on the inner side of the forearm; the handle of the ladle is fitted into the humerus bone of the upper arm. Once cemented into place, the two elements work together much like a natural elbow.

The first twenty-eight patients to receive it—twenty-four women and four men, aged forty-four to seventy-four, all with advanced rheumatoid arthritis and complete elbow joint destruction, suffering intractable pain for from three to ten years—have been relieved of pain and have regained 90 percent of normal arm function. (AM-18)

Combinations of joints. Some arthritis patients suffer from many painful and disabled joints. Not all affected joints necessarily require replacement; only those do that are very painful and no longer able to function.

When more than one joint requires replacement, priority may be given to the most painful and disabling one, and, after its replacement, one or more others may be replaced.

Sometimes other considerations are advisable. In a recent report, Dr. Alan H. Wilde, head of the section of rheumatoid surgery at Cleveland Clinic Foundation, has advised physicians: "When a patient's hip and knee joints both require total joint reconstruction, rehabilitation will be easier if the hip joint is replaced first. Once the patient has regained use of the hip, the knee joint can then be replaced. In cases of juvenile polyarthritis in which the hip and knee joints are destroyed, the hips should be replaced and the knee joints supported with long leg braces until growth is complete. Once the epiphyseal (bone) lines have closed, the knee joints can be replaced without fear of disturbing growth." (AM-19)

A simplified drug regimen for gout

Gouty arthritis is the one form of arthritis that has been most successfully attacked. Effective drugs for preventing the painful episodes in the big toe and other joints have been available for some years.

One of these drugs is allopurinol. It blocks the formation of uric acid, a chemical involved in the attacks. Allopurinol has had to be taken three times a day—a frequency that makes it difficult for some patients to use it effectively.

Now, research at the University of Pittsburgh indicates that a triple-strength tablet of allopurinol taken just once a day is effective. When gout patients were divided into two comparable groups, with one receiving the usual three tablets a day and the other taking the one larger dose once a day, the protective effect was the same. (AM-20)

An often-unsuspected cause of painful shoulder

Shoulder pain can, and very often does, have clear-cut physical causes. But in some cases, often otherwise mysterious, it may be linked with emotional problems, particularly mental depression.

Evidence comes from a recent study in Canada with fifty-six patients with shoulder pain who also were found to be suffering from depression. (Depression can be a peculiar problem, not uncommonly producing physical symptoms so troublesome that the underlying "blues" are masked by them and may not even be communicated to physicians.)

After being treated solely with antidepressant medications such as lithium carbonate and amitriptyline, forty-four of the fifty-six patients showed marked improvement in shoulder pain, with X-ray studies revealing clearing of calcification in the shoulder area.   (AM-21)

Wryneck (spasmodic torticollis)

Its cause unknown, wryneck usually appears in adulthood. Its onset may be sudden but is more likely to be gradual. Spasmodic contraction of neck muscles twists the head to one side and may bend the neck abnormally.

Difficult to treat, wryneck sometimes disappears spontaneously but more often persists for life. Some patients can help themselves, temporarily interrupting the spasm and twisting, if they exert slight pressure on the jaw on the side to which the head is being turned.

In some cases, such drugs as atropine or scopolamine may be of value. Muscle relaxing drugs are of little use but occasionally a sedative or tranquilizer has been of benefit.

Recently, one neurological study reported by Dr. G. J. Gilbert of Saint Petersburg, Florida, has indicated that a combination of drugs—amantadine hydrochloride, an agent sometimes used for Parkinsonism or shaking palsy, and haloperidol, a newer type of tranquilizer—is valuable. Benefits were obtained in every one of a group of patients receiving the combination.

Not long ago, too, a British report indicated that lithium, an antidepressant, brought improvement in at least one case, that of a thirty-six-year-old woman with a long history of depressive reactions, relieving the wryneck after failure of other medications, including amantadine and haloperidol.   (AM-22, 23)

Help for the spastic

At least some patients with disabling or painful muscle spasms, or spasticity, resulting from stroke, spinal injuries, multiple sclerosis, cerebral palsy, or other serious chronic disorders may benefit from a newer oral drug, Dantrium.

A review of experience with ten patients with weakness or paralysis resulting from stroke or spinal cord injuries or damage showed some degree of improvement in spasticity in all. Of seventeen patients with athetoid cerebral palsy, eight showed moderate improvement. Of twenty patients with multiple sclerosis, six seemed to benefit.

The drug has a tendency to produce weakness in many patients. This side effect may make little difference to a paralyzed person whose painful spasms are relieved, but can be disabling to those who could otherwise function better. (AM-24)

Shoulder dislocation: stopping repeated recurrences

Shoulders badly dislocated because of sport or other injuries can be painful. Worse yet, in some cases, repeated dislocations occur.

An operation devised a few years ago, using stainless steel staples as anchors, produced reportedly excellent results in 139 men and nine women who previously had suffered from repeated dislocations.

After the operation, performed in an hour, the shoulder is immobilized only for the first postoperative night; exercises are started on the second or third postoperative day; and patients carry out ordinary activities in three weeks, heavy work in six weeks, competitive contact sports in three months.

Drs. Harold B. Boyd and T. David Sisk of the Campbell Clinic, Memphis, Tennessee, who developed the procedure, have reported that for most patients after surgery the range of motion of the shoulder is practically normal. In their experience, patients can pass a football, pitch a baseball, use a tennis racket, and swing a golf club efficiently. (AM-25)

More recently, Drs. William Harrison, Jr., and Jerry Sisler, surgeons at Saint John's Hospital, Tulsa, Oklahoma, have reported another procedure for badly dislocated shoulders—use of a loop of Dacron, of the same kind used for synthetic blood vessels, to replace a weakened ligament.

Patients wear slings for the first ten days after the operation, then begin exercising, and by six weeks are usually back to full activity. All patients have had good results, with little pain and no recurrences of dislocations. Among the patients: a wrestler back to full competition in eight weeks. (AM-26)

CHAPTER 4
Cancer

An abnormal, purposeless, disorderly, and destructive growth, cancer is second among killer diseases, coming after heart disease. It has been and remains an extremely difficult disease to combat.

Yet some progress has been made and more is being made. Among recent advances, some could well constitute major breakthroughs.

The problem, however, increasingly is: Much of recent and current progress does not revolve around some significant new surgical technique or the development of ever more mammoth X-ray machines. Instead, it results from a multimodal approach—the bringing to bear of an array of treatment methods combined skillfully to be most effective for an individual patient.

Because that approach often requires the skills of many specialists working as a team, no individual physician or community hospital can be expected now to offer optimal care.

Certainly, still further improved treatment methods are needed. But an urgent need is for expert application of methods *already* available—and more of this shortly.

Here is a sampling of recent developments in cancer therapy which, if widely and expertly applied, promise to save the lives of many more thousands of cancer victims than are currently being saved.

Lung cancer

This has been an especially deadly malignancy. About two hundred thirty people die of it daily in the United States. Only about 8 percent of men and 12 percent of women developing lung cancer could expect to be alive five years after the diagnosis.

But a study very recently reported by Dr. Ralph E. Johnson of the National Cancer Institute indicates that a type of lung cancer that is rapidly fatal in more than 95 percent of cases now appears to be yielding to a combination of high doses of anticancer drugs and radiation.

The cancer is known as oat cell or undifferentiated small-cell carcinoma and invariably is associated with cigarette smoking.

The combination treatment involves simultaneous use of three anticancer drugs—Cytoxan, Adriamycin, and vincristine—and radiation to the tumor in the chest and to the brain where lung cancer commonly spreads. Radiation is given for three weeks, the intensive triple chemotherapy for about three months, and then all treatment is stopped.

Of the first twenty-seven patients to receive the treatment, twenty-six experienced a complete disappearance of their cancers, with twenty-one remaining free of disease after cessation of treatment for periods of up to sixteen months at the time of the report. (C-1)

Another promising development in lung cancer therapy has been reported by Dr. Jules E. Harris and other physicians at the University of Ottawa, Canada.

Surgery has been used for early lung cancer but results have been poor. In 1974, for example, Dr. C. F. Mountain of the M.D. Anderson Hospital and Tumor Institute in Houston reported that only half of five hundred seventeen patients with quite early lung cancer lived twenty-four months after surgery.

In the Ottawa study, all patients with early lung cancer received surgery and then were divided into four groups. Twelve received no further treatment. Eight received chemotherapy—high doses of an anticancer agent, methotrexate, followed by doses of citrovorum rescue factor as an antidote. Eleven patients received immunotherapy, and ten patients received a combination of the chemotherapy and immunotherapy.

The immunotherapy used in the Ottawa study consisted of a vaccine specially prepared by Dr. Ariel C. Hollinshead at George Washington University in Washington, D.C. After receiving from Ottawa specimens of surgically removed lung tumors, Dr. Hollinshead develops a specific vaccine for each patient.

In the carefully controlled comparative study, twenty-one patients who, after surgery, received immunotherapy with or without chemotherapy were found to stand a 100 percent chance of being alive thirty-six months later, compared with a 46 percent chance for patients who had surgery either alone or with chemotherapy. No patient who got both immunotherapy and chemotherapy suffered a recurrence of lung cancer.   (C-2)

Breast cancer

About 55 percent of the 89,000 women in the United States who develop breast cancer each year are found at surgery to have cancer cells in the lymph nodes surrounding the breast. Such women have had only a 45 percent chance of living for five years after operation, in contrast to an 85 percent survival rate among women without lymph node involvement.

Now early results of a study indicate that an experimental drug combination therapy can significantly reduce the recurrence of breast cancer in high-risk patients.

The study, supported by the National Cancer Institute and carried out at the Instituto Nazionale Tumori in Milan, Italy, involved 386 women who had received radical mastectomies for breast cancers in which one or more lymph nodes were affected.

One group of 179 women received no further treatment. A second group of 207, starting within two weeks after surgery, received a combination of three anticancer drugs—cyclophosphamide, methotrexate, and fluorouracil. The drugs were administered for two weeks and stopped for two weeks through twelve such cycles. The drugs are potent; they produced side effects in some women—nausea, appetite loss, hair loss (never complete and with regrowth occurring before the end of treatment).

But in the drug-treated group for periods of up to twenty-seven months, only 5.3 percent of the women have developed cancer recurrences as against 24 percent of the women who received no treatment after surgery.

Meanwhile, in the United States as well, studies have been going on with postsurgery therapies including single drugs, two-drug combinations, and combinations of drugs with immunotherapy or hormone therapy. For example, a single drug, L-PAM, has been found to reduce cancer recurrence from 22 percent to 9 percent two years after surgery. It is expected that out of such studies will come data to suggest the most effective postoperative therapy producing the least serious side effects and greatest saving of life.

Inasmuch, however, as all studies thus far show a clear advantage of postoperative drug treatment, experts are suggesting that physicians start using it for all breast cancer patients with cancerous lymph nodes.   (C-3)

Leukemia

Acute lymphocytic leukemia (ALL), the most frequent form of childhood cancer, was considered almost uniformly fatal only a decade ago.

One of the first valuable developments was use of such drugs as prednisone and vincristine sulfate to induce remission. Then, multiple drugs were administered for two to three years in efforts to eliminate the disease. With the discovery that the major form of initial relapse, arachnoid leukemia, could be prevented by irradiation in the first month of remission, about one half of the children so treated have remained free of all evidence of leukemia, and about 80 percent of these children have remained free of leukemia after all treatment has been stopped for periods now of up to ten years. This suggests that most are cured.   (C-4)

Hodgkin's disease

At one time, this cancer of the lymph system, which can affect lymph nodes, spleen, and lymphoid tissue, generally was 75 percent fatal.

Recently, however, the use of radiation therapy along with combination chemotherapy (involving varied anticancer drugs) has led to long-term survival and possible cure in more than 80 percent of patients, including children and adolescents as well as adults. Even many with advanced, widely disseminated disease are responding.
(C-4)

Rhabdomyosarcoma

Embryonal rhabdomyosarcoma, a muscle tumor of children, once had a dismal outlook. Radical surgery to remove the tumor often was followed by recurrence near the original site or at distant points in the body. Radiotherapy produced only temporary partial regressions.

Then a combination of three drugs—dactinomycin, cyclophosphamide, and vincristine—was found to reduce tumors in most children, and it became reasonable to use the drug combination to supplement surgery and radiotherapy.

Other findings followed. When the three-drug combination was used before surgery, it shrank the tumor enough to allow complete removal by less radical surgery, avoiding amputations in many cases. It also turned out that when the drugs were administered together with radiotherapy, more prompt and complete tumor regression occurred. And, finally, when the drugs were given for one to two years after surgery, radiotherapy or both, they cut the risk of spread of the cancer.

Today, almost half of children receiving coordinated therapy with surgery, irradiation, and combination drugs can be expected to survive free of tumor, a 400 percent improvement over past experience.   (C-4)

Bone cancers

Ewing's sarcoma, a highly malignant tumor of bone that strikes children and young adults, has been one of the most deadly cancers. At best, in the past, only five to ten patients in one hundred could expect to survive five years.

Now intensive treatment, combining high-dose radiation, anticancer drugs (Adriamycin, Cytoxan, and vincristine), prophylactic radiation to the brain, and intraspinal injection of methotrexate, is saving 50 percent of patients, report Drs. Thomas C. Pomery and Ralph E. Johnson of the National Cancer Institute.   (C-5)

Osteogenic sarcoma, a bone cancer that has been most resistant to treatment, strikes teen-agers and preteen-agers in the arms and legs. Even after amputation, one half of patients have had spread of cancer to the lungs within six months and 85 percent within two years, commonly followed within months thereafter by death.

But within the past two years, studies at Children's Cancer Research Foundation, Boston, and elsewhere have indicated that chemotherapy following amputation is changing the picture. For example, of a group of children and young adults treated with Adriamycin, cyclophosphamide, and methotrexate in monthly cycles for ten months, better than 85 percent are surviving free of tumor for up to twenty-four months thus far.

Other cancers

The likelihood that Wilms' tumor, a kidney cancer and one of the most common malignancies of childhood, can be cured has increased markedly in recent years as the result of vigorous treatment combining surgery, postoperative irradiation, and combination chemotherapy. In one study, at the Princess Margaret Hospital, Toronto, for example, the five-year survival rate increased from 54 percent for children diagnosed from 1960 to 1965 to 81 percent for those diagnosed since 1966, because of increased ability to cure metastatic disease (spread of the cancer beyond the kidney) with intensive multimodal therapy.   (C-6)

Some improvement has occurred in the outlook for patients with cancer of the colon and rectum with the finding in an extensive Veterans Administration study that with use of X-ray treatment before surgery, 40.8 percent of patients are living five years or more compared with 28.4 percent of those not irradiated.   (C-7)

Currently, because of the notable improvement brought about, in some of the cancers already mentioned, by use of drug therapy combined with other methods of treatment, postsurgical chemotherapy is being studied for its lifesaving value in other cancers, including those of the ovary, colon, prostate, and bladder, where the likelihood of recurrence is high.

What to do if cancer strikes in your family

Officials of the National Cancer Institute, cancer experts at major medical centers, and researchers who are opening up new pathways to improved cancer treatment are increasingly concerned—and now becoming more and more forthrightly vocal—about the poor delivery of cancer care.

They point to these problems:

The vast majority—80 percent or more—of patients with cancer are first seen by a local internist, pediatrician, or family physician who has had no formal training in treating cancer. Most medical schools give no intensive courses in diagnosis and treatment of cancer.

To make matters worse, many local doctors hesitate to refer their cancer patients to cancer specialists, for one thing, because it reflects, or so they think, on their ability and, for another, because many still feel that almost all cancers are incurable.

Not long ago, Dr. Vincent T. DeVita, Jr., director of the National Cancer Institute division of cancer treatment, declared that "the phrase, 'Let them die with dignity,' is too often used when the patient could have years of useful life or a normal lifetime."

Some 85 percent of cancer patients go to community hospitals that commonly lack trained personnel—physicians, nurses, technicians—and all the necessary equipment for optimum handling of cancer.

Efforts now are being made to improve diagnosis and treatment of cancer.

Directed to do so by Congress, the National Cancer Institute, going beyond research functions, has developed seventeen comprehensive cancer centers across the country. These centers serve several functions. They study new cancer therapies and try them for patients who cannot be helped in any other way. They expertly apply the latest established treatments. Some operate programs to instruct, without charge, physicians on cancer advances and also teach hospitals in their areas how to improve cancer care. (You can obtain the name and address of the comprehensive center nearest you by writing to the Office of Cancer Communications, National Cancer Institute, Building 31, Room 10 A 30, Bethesda, Md. 20014.)

When it comes to children's cancer, there is now a good network of centers—cancer hospitals that treat many children and pediatric hospitals that see a lot of childhood cancer—capable of providing expert care. They include Children's Hospital of Boston, Children's Hospital of Philadelphia, Children's Hospital of Los Angeles, Children's Hospital of Denver, Children's Hospital of Columbus, Children's Orthopedic of Seattle, Roswell Park Memorial Institute in Buffalo, Saint Jude Children's Research Hospital in Memphis, Stanford Medical Center's Children's Hospital in Palo Alto, California, Memorial Hospital in New York City, and M. D. Anderson Hospital and Tumor Institute in Houston. There are also many university hospitals across the country with excellent departments of pediatrics, staffed with pediatric surgeons, radiation therapists, and other specialists skilled in treating childhood cancer. And there are major metropolitan hospitals and large private institutions such as the Mayo Clinic where excellent care may be obtained.

To protect yourself against both misdiagnosis and poor treatment, experts urge that you always get a second opinion and never accept the word of just one physician.

It's advisable, many experts say, to not let your family physician pick your consultant. He may or may not know the proper one. You can call the nearest medical school or the American Cancer Society and get the name of a cancer specialist.

CHAPTER 5

Ear Disorders

Vertigo (dizziness)

Virtually everyone has experienced the sensation of dizziness as the result of whirling around too rapidly or too long or perhaps while looking down from a great height. This mild sensation is markedly different from true vertigo.

With true vertigo, there is a sensation of being whirled about in space or of objects whirling about the sufferer. Often vertigo is accompanied by nausea, pallor, sweating.

The possible causes for vertigo are many since it involves a disturbance of the equilibratory or balancing apparatus—and that apparatus consists of the labyrinth of the inner ear, areas of the brain, the eye, and the sensory nerves of muscles, joints, and tendons. Any of a wide variety of disorders may affect one or more of these balancing apparatus components.

Vertigo may thus stem from infections or inflammations in or around the middle ear, obstruction of the ear canal or of the eustachian tube leading from throat to ear, or Menière's disease (see below). General infections may cause vertigo that may persist after the acute stages of the infections have passed. Medications such as quinine, salicylates (aspirin and aspirinlike compounds), and streptomycin may set off vertigo; so, on occasion, may alcohol, caffeine, nicotine, and various sedatives. Eye problems such as glaucoma or ocular imbalance may be involved. Among many other possible causes: anemia, high blood pressure, and, less frequently, brain tumors.

Relief of vertigo depends on determining and eliminating the cause. Symptomatic treatment may include use of a tranquilizing agent such as perphenazine or an antihistamine such as dimenhydrinate, which has a depressant effect on an overstimulated labyrinth.

More recently, another antihistamine, meclizine hydrochloride, has proved effective in many cases in providing symptomatic relief. Studies at the Mount Sinai School of Medicine, New York City, have found it to be valuable in reducing both the severity and frequency of vertigo attacks and in ameliorating such vertigo-associated symptoms as nausea, postural instability, and involuntary eye movements. (EA-1)

Vertigo plus hearing impairment (Menière's disease)

Menière's disease, which involves a disturbance in the labyrinth of the inner ear, produces recurrent attacks of vertigo, nausea, hearing impairment, and ringing in the ears (tinnitus). Attacks last from a few minutes to several hours. The course may vary. Sometimes the vertigo attacks stop but the hearing impairment and tinnitus continue. Or the vertigo may stop only when deafness is complete.

Many medications have been used to treat or help prevent attacks; no one is effective in all cases. The medications include antihistamines, diuretic agents to help reduce fluid accumulations, agents such as niacin and nicotinyl alcohol to help expand blood vessels and improve blood flow. For a severe acute attack, an injection of atropine or scopolamine may provide relief.

In severe incapacitating cases, surgical treatment has been used. If the labyrinth disturbance is diagnosed as affecting only one ear and useful hearing in that ear is lacking, electrical coagulation of the labyrinth has been helpful. Good results in many cases also have been obtained with the use of high frequency sound waves (ultrasound) to selectively destroy the labyrinth while preserving the hearing apparatus.

Recently, some new approaches to medical treatment of Menière's disease have been reported.

A new diuretic treatment. Swedish physicians at the Akademiska Sjokhuset in Uppsala have reported promising results with chlorthalidone, a diuretic. Their work started with a group of thirty-four patients treated with the drug and followed for seven years. Improvement was experienced by twenty-four, with the most pronounced benefit being reduced prevalence and intensity of vertigo.

The drug also was tried in 220 severely incapacitated patients who had been hospitalized for possible surgery. In 133, improvement following use of the drug was sufficient to avoid need for operation.

The Swedish physicians report that they have no evidence that chlorthalidone arrests the course of the disease, but it does in some cases appear to reduce need for surgery and may help patients, when it is successful, to lead an active life.   (EA-2)

Lithium treatment. Lithium carbonate is a drug often used to treat manic-depressive illness. At the University of Copenhagen, Denmark, Dr. Ole Rafaelson has studied its use in Menière's disease.

Of forty patients for whom it was tried, ten discontinued its use quickly because of a side effect such as weight gain. Of the other thirty, twenty-one found the drug valuable. Sixteen of the twenty-one remain on lithium. Five could stop all treatment after ten to eighteen months with complete elimination of Menière's symptoms.

Weight gain is a common, even though not invariable, side effect of lithium treatment. The usual gain is eleven to twenty-two pounds. pounds.   (EA-3)

Food allergy and Menière's. Is it possible that in some cases Menière's disease is due to food allergies and that symptoms disappear when offending foods are avoided?

So Dr. Jack D. Clemis of Northwestern University Medical School, Chicago, has reported.

The food groups most commonly responsible are wheat, corn, eggs, and milk.

Dr. Clemis has found that detection of specific food allergies is simplified by use of a test developed by Dr. William T. K. Bryan of Washington University, Saint Louis. Using the white cells from a small sample of blood, some seventy common food allergens can be tested. If there is allergy to a specific food, the white cells disintegrate when the food is added to the sample.

Among patients reported by Dr. Clemis: A fifty-five-year-old surgeon faced with early retirement because of vertigo and hearing loss. Surgery on the labyrinth in the right ear had provided relief for three months. But then hearing fluctuations increased in severity, tinnitus persisted on the right side and occurred intermittently on the left, ear fullness and pressure developed, and there were episodes of imbalance.

The blood test showed a whole series of allergies—to oats, rice, barley, safflower, cottonseed, milk, eggs, tuna, shrimp, crab, herring, mustard, tomatoes, cane sugar, coffee, bananas, cantaloupe, yeast, soy, almonds, and peanuts.

During six weeks on an elimination diet, the surgeon lost fifteen pounds but had a marked gain in hearing, although some fluctuations in the hearing persisted. After three months, his hearing was back to virtually normal levels in his left ear and other symptoms were relieved.

Once foods are removed from the diet, Dr. Clemis has found, they can usually be reintroduced in small quantities beginning about a month after all symptoms have cleared, although it's unlikely a patient can eat them ever again in as great a proportion as before Menière's disease developed.   (EA-4)

Reducing high blood-fat levels to help inner ear disease. A reduction by diet of high blood levels of cholesterol and triglycerides (fats) may, it appears, help some sufferers from Menière's disease and similar inner ear disturbances producing hearing loss and vertigo.

High levels of cholesterol and triglycerides have, of course, been linked to atherosclerosis, the artery-clogging disease that leads to heart attacks. A first clue to the possible role of elevated blood-fat levels in some hearing problems came several years ago when Dr. Samuel Rosen, a distinguished New York ear specialist, surveyed hearing loss in many parts of the world and discovered that wherever there was a high incidence of elevated cholesterol, atherosclerosis, and heart disease, hearing levels tended to be reduced.

It seemed to Rosen that atherosclerosis might in fact sometimes first affect the delicate inner ear hearing structures, and hearing loss might even be a first indication of atherosclerosis in some cases. Rosen had proposed a provocative question: Might a reversal in diet bring about a reversal in hearing loss?

It remained for Dr. James T. Spencer, a Charleston, West Virginia, ear specialist, himself a victim of hearing loss and vertigo, to determine that it could.

In July 1971, Spencer had become increasingly concerned about his own health. For five years, he had suffered progressive loss of hearing with periods of vertigo. In addition, allergy problems were causing discomfort. Aware that he was sensitive to wheat, he decided to eliminate wheat from his diet.

Over the next few weeks, eating no wheat items, he lost a few pounds, felt a bit better, but was far from well. At that point, he had some laboratory tests done. They showed elevated levels of cholesterol and triglycerides. Whereupon he went on a diet that eliminated refined sugar, kept total carbohydrate (sugars and starches) low, and increased intake of protein with minimal saturated fat.

In addition to losing another fourteen pounds, he also found his blood-fat levels dropping markedly. Within three months, to his astonishment, he found that he had regained 87 percent of his lost hearing.

It was while pondering why a diet designed to lower blood-fat levels and reduce risk of atherosclerosis could have had any influence on hearing that he recalled the findings and suggestion of Dr. Rosen.

Soon afterward, he saw as a patient an ex-Marine who had been medically discharged because of hearing loss, vertigo, and ringing of the ears that had persisted for four years despite repeated hospitalizations and study.

The man had a maddening roaring in his right ear, a severe sixty-decibel loss of hearing in the same ear, a thirty-decibel loss in the other ear, was having frequent attacks of vertigo with nausea and vomiting, was overweight, and had excessively high blood-fat levels.

Within five weeks after being placed on the diet Spencer had used for himself, the ex-Marine had a twelve-decibel gain in his right ear. After another two weeks, he had lost twenty-five pounds and reported some improvement of hearing in both ears. After still another month, he had lost ten pounds more and his hearing acuity increased further.

Within three years during which he saw 444 patients with inner ear problems, Spencer found that 207, or 46.6 percent, had hyperlipoproteinemia (high blood-fat levels), another forty-six, or 10.3 percent, were borderline.

Symptoms were varied. Many had hearing loss mainly in one ear with some deterioration in the other ear. Many also experienced noises in the ear, fullness, or pain. Some were subject to acute vertigo attacks. In some cases, headaches were a problem as well. Many patients were overweight to some degree; some were obese.

Spencer fitted diets to individual patients. Hyperlipoproteinemia takes several forms: marked elevation of blood cholesterol alone; marked triglyceride elevation alone; or elevation of both.

Essential diet features included reduction of cholesterol intake, reduction or elimination of saturated fats and increases in polyunsaturated, controlled carbohydrate intake, elimination of sugars and concentrated sweets—with greater or lesser emphasis on one or more features depending upon the individual patient.

Most of the patients have benefited, Spencer has reported. Hearing loss has been stopped and in some cases gains of as much as thirty decibels in an affected ear have been achieved. Acute vertigo attacks have stopped in some cases, become much less frequent and severe in others. Headaches, pressure in the head, and fullness in the ears have been among the first symptoms to be relieved. Blood-fat levels have been brought down and weight has been lost.

There should be no problems, Spencer advises, for physicians interested in testing for hyperlipoproteinemia in patients with hearing problems. Many laboratories do the testing, which requires only a small sample of blood.

Physicians also can obtain a handbook for physicians entitled *The Dietary Management of Hyperlipoproteinemia* from the Office of Heart and Lung Information, National Heart and Lung Institute, Bethesda, Md. 20014. The handbook defines the specific diet for each type of hyperlipoproteinemia. Copies of diets are also available for physicians to give to patients.   (EA-5)

Controlling fluctuant hearing loss

Fullness and ringing of the ears, fluctuation in hearing, and vertigo occur in an inner-ear disorder called fluctuant hearing loss—and the four manifestations usually appear in that order. The disorder usually occurs in middle age, affects both sexes equally and, not infrequently, both ears.

Abnormal retention of fluids in the inner ear is known to be involved. The disorder can stem from many causes including diabetes, syphilis, excessive blood levels of fat, excessive smoking, high salt intake, and even anxiety.

At the Memphis (Tennessee) Otologic Clinic, Drs. J. J. Shea and

A. E. Kitabchi have found abnormal glucose tolerance, indicative of latent diabetes, present in 57 percent of cases and in 50 percent the intolerance had not been previously detected. Excessive smoking was next in order of frequency (10 percent), followed by other factors such as high blood-fat levels, allergy, and anxiety (each 7 percent).

Correction of any abnormality such as diabetes can be helpful; elimination of smoking can also be helpful.

And frequently, the two investigators report, the disorder can be managed by treatment that includes a low-salt diet, use of a potassium-sparing diuretic such as Dyazide (a drug to eliminate excess fluids without causing loss of potassium from the body), and inhalation of a mixture of oxygen and carbon dioxide to dilate blood vessels in the inner ear and promote circulation.

Additionally, when warranted in individual patients, a low-carbohydrate, low-calorie diet is used to control glucose intolerance; a low-fat diet is used for those with elevated blood-fat levels; elimination of allergy-producing agents if possible or use of an antihistamine, cyproheptadine, is prescribed in those with allergy; and birth-control and diet pills (both suspected of causing fluctuant hearing loss) are stopped in those taking them.

Such treatment, Drs. Shea and Kitabchi report, has produced good results in preserving hearing and controlling dizziness.   (EA-6)

Fluoride for hearing loss in young adults

One of the most common causes of progressive hearing loss in young adults is a softening of the bones in the inner and middle ear. Originally called otosclerosis but more recently otospongiosis, the softening affects about 1 percent of Americans, is more common among women, usually above the age of twenty and most often between twenty-five and forty-five. It usually affects both ears within two years of onset and is a hereditary disorder.

As soft, spongelike bone replaces the normal ivory-hard bone, the tiny bones in the ear, which normally vibrate to transmit sound waves, no longer do so.

Recently, Dr. George E. Shambaugh, Jr., of Northwestern University Medical School, Chicago, has reported that sodium fluoride, the same compound used to help harden children's teeth, has proved valuable for about 80 percent of patients. Similar results have been reported by Dr. Jean Causse of Béziers, France, in an equal number of patients. And still more recently, Dr. Frederick H. Linthicum, Jr., of the Ear Research Institute in Los Angeles has confirmed their findings.

The treatment usually consists of 0.5 gram of calcium gluconate before a meal and 20 milligrams of sodium fluoride after each of two meals a day, supplemented with one multivitamin tablet once a day to supply, among other things, 400 units of vitamin D to help intestinal absorption of calcium.

Is it dangerous to take that much fluoride? Does it accumulate in the body and cause serious side effects? Dr. Shambaugh reports that exhaustive tests have not turned up any evidence that the doses of fluoride harm any body organ.

The major value of treatment is prevention of further hearing loss, but a few patients have experienced small improvements in hearing.

(EA-7)

Acupuncture, electrostimulation, and hearing

Does acupuncture have any remarkable value for improving hearing? After many conflicting reports, one of the latest, announced by the American Academy of Pediatrics, indicates that when Vanderbilt University and Central Michigan University investigators checked on 111 patients who had undergone acupuncture treatment, they found that only 4 percent showed some improvement while an equal proportion showed a decrease in hearing.

Another method of treatment, "transdermal electrostimulation," which involves electrical stimulation through electrodes across the head, has been under study since 1969 but thus far does not appear to be effective.

Conclude the investigators: Neither acupuncture nor transdermal stimulation can be dismissed completely; either or both, with further research, may prove to have some usefulness; but no evidence presently exists warranting the use of either for the hearing-impaired.

(EA-8)

Hearing aids: even the best can vary greatly in effectiveness for an individual user

In a study by Dr. O. Haug and other Houston investigators with 298 patients, investigators selected hearing aids, several for each patient, that theoretically, on the basis of the characteristics of the aids and the needs of the patients, should have provided peak performance.

But, in actual use, there were marked differences in effectiveness. In almost half (47 percent) of the patients, there were differences of 20 percent or more in speech discrimination between what proved to be for them the poorest and best performing aids. In 86 percent of the patients, there were differences of 10 percent or more.

Such considerable differences, the study suggests, justify the effort and expense involved in carefully evaluating various aids for an individual patient rather than letting it go at merely choosing an aid that theoretically should be suitable.   (EA-9)

A simple solution for ear wax cleaning

The hazards of historic methods of cleaning out ear wax—with toothpicks, paper clips, even cotton swabs—are substantial. The danger of eardrum puncture and hearing loss is enough to make doctors leery about using forceps or other mechanical devices.

In one study at the University of Pennsylvania Medical School, Philadelphia, with twenty-seven patients with self-induced eardrum punctures, thirteen were found to be caused by commercially available cotton-tipped sticks, four by bobby pins, others by sticks, combs, and metal instruments. Such punctures are serious and best treated by surgery within twenty-four hours to repair the drum and, if necessary, to realign any fractured or dislocated bones of hearing in the middle ear.

The University of Pennsylvania investigators urge that no cleaning be done deep in the ear canal, noting that it isn't necessary, anyhow, because the ear has a self-cleaning mechanism. When wax appears on the outside, it can be removed with a soft paper or cloth towel. (EA-10)

Another study indicates that when excessive, obstructive hard ear wax is present, a single application of a liquid preparation, Cerumenex, is effective. While several preparations to be applied by dropper have been available before, they have usually required three or more applications. The study—by Drs. Arshad Amjad and Alan A. Scheer of the New York Foundation for Otologic Research, New York City—found that one application of Cerumenex was enough to clear hard wax obstruction in as many as 96 percent of cases. In only one instance was there a side effect—mild reddening of the ear canal.   (EA-11)

Coughing from just a hair in the ear

Although it may seem unlikely—and, because it does, may go unsuspected—one possible cause of chronic coughing can be a hair in the ear that touches the eardrum.

The coughing mechanism—which is designed to remove any irritating substances in the breathing passages—is triggered by a message about the irritation to the cough center in the brain, which then sends out another message to produce the coughing response.

But Drs. Allan P. Wolff, Mark May, and Douglas Nuelle of Washington University School of Medicine, Saint Louis, report that a hair touching the eardrum can also lead to a message about irritation, putting the cough center into action and keeping it in action so that coughing can become a chronic problem until the hair is removed. Several patients, they note, have been cured of chronic cough simply by removal of a hair.   (EA-12)

A serious risk in ear-lobe piercing—and how to avoid it

A recent finding is that instruments used to pierce the ears, if not properly sterilized, can transmit the serious liver disease hepatitis—and may in fact be an important route for hepatitis spread in the United States.

The finding comes from a study begun in the Seattle, Washington, area when one hepatitis victim noted that her ears had been pierced in a jewelry store and the jeweler had used instruments soaked in an alcohol solution between piercings. Alcohol does not destroy the hepatitis virus. Investigators soon were able to trace hepatitis in seven other young women to ear-lobe piercing. Further study established that even some physicians doing ear piercing were using an ineffective cleansing solution for instruments.

Urge the investigators: either single-use disposable instruments should be used or the instruments must be sterilized in an autoclave or boiled for twenty minutes to destroy the hepatitis virus.   (EA-13)

Simplified surgery for correcting prominent ears

Prominent ears, including those that stick straight out from the head, now can be corrected by a simple new operative technique.

Developed by a Viennese plastic surgeon, Dr. Hans G. Bruck, and reported in detail here to United States ear specialists and surgeons, the operation, which has been used successfully in more than three hundred fifty patients in Vienna since 1968, is performed under local anesthesia and does not require an overnight hospital stay.

Unlike previous operations that sometimes interfered with full blood flow to the ears, the new technique does not—which may be a matter of importance in cold regions where ear frostbite is a hazard.

The technique requires no special instruments and can be learned quickly by experienced otolaryngologists and plastic surgeons. Although ideally done at about the age of five or six, it also is effective for adults, according to Dr. Bruck.   (EA-14)

CHAPTER 6

Emotional/Behavioral Problems

Depression: the most common psychologic ill

Virtually everyone at one time or another experiences mental depression. It commonly follows loss or separation from a familiar person or place and brings with it feelings of helplessness and hopelessness that in a relatively short time normally subside spontaneously.

But in some people depression escalates to a serious condition. It is now recognized to be the most common of all psychologic ills. Fortunately, it is one that often can be relieved readily by treatment.

A National Institute of Mental Health survey indicates that as many as eight million people a year suffer depression severe enough to merit treatment.

But depression can be sneaky; it often wears disguises. Some studies have indicated that the elapsed time from onset of symptoms to accurate recognition of depression ranges up to as long as thirty-six months, during which patients often, if they receive any treatment at all, may be treated for other illnesses.　　　　　(EB-1)

Depression: recognizing guises and disguises

In serious depression, there is a sustained, chronic change of mood, an extended lowering of the spirits.

A virtually universal symptom is loss of enjoyment of things and activities that under normal circumstances make life worth living.

Among other major reactions that may be experienced are the following (it is unusual for all to be present in a particular case):

Difficulty in concentration, perhaps indicated by reading a book or even a newspaper, or watching a TV program, only to discover that nothing of what was read or seen is retained.

Fatigue, with easy tiring and lack of drive to do things and get things done.

Sleeping difficulty, particularly a tendency to wake up early feeling exhausted (and depressed).

Remorse over not having done things you should have done or having done what you should not have done.

Guilt, with feelings of being unfair to family, friends, and others.

Indecision about important matters and even at times about the most simple things.

Reduced sexual activity.

General loss of interest, with indifference to people, things, and ideas once of importance to you.

Irritability and impatience over even trivial matters.

Suicidal thoughts.   (EB-2)

In addition, there may be other—physical—symptoms and, not infrequently, these may so overshadow "blue" feelings that attention concentrates on them; patients seeking medical help often do so for the physical problems without revealing the others that would provide clues to the presence of depression.

Headaches are common in depression, occurring in as many as four-fifths of patients as a major complaint, and in some cases the only complaint. Depressive headaches do not have a favorite site but do tend to be worse in the morning than in the evening and often stubbornly resist the usual headache remedies.

Loss of appetite is frequent. Gastrointestinal symptoms can be diverse. Depression often is responsible for complaints of gas and for abdominal pains unexplained by physical findings. Some depressed people suffer severely from digestive upsets, nausea, vomiting, constipation, or diarrhea and may be mistakenly thought to have ulcers or colitis.

Depression may also cause urinary frequency or urgency, sometimes accompanied by burning and pressure sensations in the bladder area.

Some of the depressed experience heart palpitations, chest constriction, and pain in the area of the heart and may believe they have heart disease.

Others may experience visual disturbances, ear noises, mouth dryness, numbness or tingling sensations, and skin blotches.

A British study, among others, has shown that some of the depressed experience difficulty in breathing that may arouse fears of lung cancer or emphysema.

Such physical disturbances have come to be called the "somatic mask of depression." They often can be relieved effectively with antidepressant medication.

Increasing attention also is being paid to depression in the elderly which may appear not as a mood change but as confusion, disorientation, agitation, memory loss, and may be considered to be dementia when in reality it is not and will respond to antidepressant medication.   (EB-3)

Depression: effective treatments

A considerable variety of antidepressant medications is available today. Among them are such agents as imipramine (trade named Tofranil); desipramine (trade named Elavil); protriptyline (trade named Vivactil); nortriptyline (trade named Aventyl); doxepin (trade named Sinequan); and amitriptyline plus perphenazine (trade named Triavil and Etraton).

Commonly, an antidepressant can be found that is suitable for the individual patient.

There is some controversy among psychiatrists about whether drug treatment cures depression or only relieves the symptoms. Some psychiatrists believe that psychotherapy is essential for cure. Others consider that drugs go beyond relieving symptoms and help to correct basic malfunctions. They admit that depressives, like virtually everybody else, have psychological problems and like everybody else might, ideally, benefit to some degree from psychotherapy. But that is not possible, and psychotherapy should be reserved for those in whom neurosis is a serious factor in the depression. They also note that in their experience quite often patients find that when depression clears up with drug therapy, most of the other problems also disappear, i.e., become more manageable and normal instead of overwhelming.

An added aid. It now appears that for some patients who do not respond adequately to antidepressant medication, the addition of thyroid hormone to treatment may bring dramatic improvement.

In one study by Dr. F. E. Goodwin of the National Institute of Mental Health with twenty-five patients not responding well to antidepressants, fourteen improved when twenty-five micrograms of T3, a thyroid hormone, was added to treatment. In some cases the improvement was startlingly rapid—occurring within a few hours—but the average was five and a half days.   (EB-4)

In another study, also reported by Dr. Goodwin of the National Institute of Mental Health, Bethesda, Maryland, 75 percent of a group of patients who had been unresponsive to standard antidepressant drugs such as Tofranil and Elavil improved rapidly when T3 was added in doses of twenty-five micrograms. The hormone was effective, Dr. Goodwin found, even though all those benefiting had apparently normal thyroid function.   (EB-5)

Manic depressive illness and lithium

When depressive illness is in one direction—down—it is called unipolar. But manic or bipolar depression affects an estimated four million Americans who suffer recurrent bouts of severe depression alternating with manic behavior—episodes of great elation that in some cases may be manifested in flamboyant speech and action, or feelings of being unable to do any wrong.

Treatment of manic-depressive patients has been discouraging. When depressed, they may respond to antidepressant drugs. For the manic state, two main methods of treatment have been electroshock and heavy doses of powerful tranquilizers. Neither has been entirely satisfactory. Tranquilizers have a sedative effect, subduing patients, keeping them in a kind of chemical straitjacket until a manic episode is over. Electroshock has produced only temporary benefit. About 75 percent of bipolar depression victims have had repeated recurrences.

It is into this therapy gap that a drug with a checkered history has stepped. Lithium was first discovered as an element in nature in 1817, but there is some evidence that it may have been used unknowingly long before as a treatment. The fifth century Roman physician Caelius Aurelianus recommended use of alkaline spring waters, which were probably high in lithium content, for treatment of mania.

Toward the end of the nineteenth century, lithium salts seemed to work to break up kidney stones in laboratory test tubes, but, when tried on patients, proved valueless. Then in the late 1940s, lithium in the form of its chloride salt became a popular salt substitute for patients on low-sodium diets. What was not known was that lithium may be dangerous for patients with congestive heart disease and associated kidney disease, and when four deaths and many serious but nonlethal poisonings were attributed to lithium chloride, the drug was taken off the market in 1949.

But that same year, an Australian psychiatrist, Dr. John Cade, was first discovering the value of another lithium compound—lithium carbonate—in bipolar depression. When he gave the drug to ten manic depressives during the manic phase of their illness, all responded and within one to two weeks were exhibiting normal or near-normal behavior.

Other Australian investigators began to find the drug valuable in small-scale studies. By 1967, two Danish doctors, Mogens Schou and Poul Baastrup, after studying use of lithium carbonate in hundreds of patients, could report that "lithium is the first drug demonstrated as a clearcut prophylactic agent against one of the major psychoses."

Within a few years successful studies were being reported in the United States, and the FDA approved the drug for use in treating manic-depressive illness.

For a patient in an acute manic state, lithium usually can control the manic behavior, but initial improvement may require five to ten days. If a patient is extremely manic, many psychiatrists start with a tranquilizer such as haloperidol or chlorpromazine to get quick control until the lithium has a chance to become effective. Mildly disturbed patients may be treated with lithium alone.

The drug appears to normalize a patient by getting at the underlying chemical problem in manic-depressive illness, thus shortening the episode, and also leaving the patient feeling less drugged. Its greatest value is its effectiveness in preventing recurrences not only of the mania but also of the depression. While large doses may be required for controlling acute mania, afterward, lower maintenance doses are used prophylactically.

While on a maintenance dose, a patient may begin to note some of the changes such as mild restlessness, insomnia, and overactivity that heralded previous manic episodes. But now these serve as alerts, and an increase in the lithium dosage usually aborts the symptoms and prevents a manic episode.

The drug is also valuable in preventing many depressive attacks. It is of no use for overcoming depression once present; at that point, an antidepressant drug is needed. But on lithium maintenance, depressive incidents are less frequent and less intense and those that occur are more readily and quickly overcome with addition of an antidepressant drug.

More recently, studies have been indicating that lithium may be valuable in some cases of recurrent unipolar depression. Although it does not always eliminate recurrences, it frequently reduces their frequency and severity.

Psychiatrists and other physicians in private practice now are using lithium treatment in suitable patients. Some lithium clinics are operating. At the Lithium Clinic of the New York State Psychiatric Institute in New York City, where research has been going on for many years and more than a thousand patients have been treated, lithium maintenance therapy is simple.

At the clinic, new patients are seen once a week until they are stabilized on lithium and clinically well. Then they return every four weeks for evaluation, behavior and mood ratings, and monitoring of blood lithium levels, with trained non-physician personnel doing much of the work. A psychiatrist is called only if a patient is experiencing mood changes or possible side reactions from lithium.

In one recent study at the clinic, a group of patients, each of whom had had at least two manic-depressive episodes in two years before entering the clinic, were followed for eighteen months during which they remained free of trouble and never required the direct services of a psychiatrist.

At least one expert, Dr. Ronald R. Fieve, chief of Psychiatric Research at the Clinic of the New York State Psychiatric Institute, believes that lithium is not being as widely used as it should be; that where millions could benefit, only some one hundred thousand or fewer are being treated; that many physicians and hospitals are still needlessly continuing to use electroshock therapy and multiple drug therapies. Fieve also believes that as many as 30 percent of schizophrenics in mental hospitals may not be schizophrenics at all but unrecognized victims of manic-depressive illness. He advocates an intensive educational campaign for physicians as well as the lay public.

As for the public, Fieve says, anyone who finds his or her social, sexual, or vocational life disturbed by a mood swing should consider that depression may be at work. The family physician then should be consulted and told what the patient thinks he or she has, and, if necessary, there should be insistence that the physician consider it seriously and do something about it, perhaps making a referral to the nearest expert in diagnosing and treating depressive disorders. If lithium treatment is indicated, once it has been started and the right dosage established, it is likely that the family physician can take over, seeing the patient occasionally and carrying out simple periodic blood tests to make certain that all is going well.   (EB-6)

Lithium for a character disorder

A psychiatric diagnosis, "emotionally unstable character disorder," is applied to people with maladaptive behavior. They may be given to truancy, have poor job histories, and have difficulty accepting reasonable authority. They also tend to have great swings of mood, from feelings of depression to excessive elation unrelated to reality.

At Hillside Hospital, Glen Oaks, New York, a team of psychiatrists studying use of lithium carbonate in a group of twenty-one such patients have reported that it is valuable in its ability to decrease the mood swings that often trigger the behavioral problems, and appears to be superior to any previous treatment.   (EB-7)

Propranolol for schizophrenia

Propranolol, a drug often used for anginal chest pain and other heart problems, appears to be helpful for at least a few patients with schizophrenia, according to a British study.

At Friern Hospital, London, fourteen patients who had not responded to usual tranquilizing agents were given propranolol. In six, all symptoms remitted completely. Five others showed moderate to marked improvement. In the six with complete remissions, improvement began within a few days of start of the treatment and all have remained well for up to six months thus far on a daily dose of the drug.   (EB-8)

Caffeinism as a readily correctable, but overlooked, cause of anxiety

Excessive caffeine intake—not only via coffee and tea but also via cola drinks, hot chocolate, cocoa, and chocolate bars and, too, caffeine-containing medications—can produce symptoms very much like those of a worrisome psychiatric disorder, chronic anxiety.

The symptoms include restlessness, irritability, insomnia, headaches, muscle twitching and, occasionally, vomiting and diarrhea.

Also, patients unaware of any particularly heavy caffeine intake may be treated unsuccessfully with tranquilizers and other drugs when the need is not to add new drugs but to cut the intake of the responsible drug, caffeine.

At the Walter Reed Army Medical Center, Dr. John F. Greden, then director of psychiatric research there and now on the faculty of the University of Michigan School of Medicine, uncovered cases of caffeinism. Among them: a nurse who, after acquiring a new coffeemaker, had begun to drink ten to twelve cups of strong coffee daily; an army colonel who drank as many as fourteen cups of coffee daily plus cocoa and colas; a sergeant proud of the fact that he drank "more coffee than anybody in the office" along with tea and cola.

In each case, there were such symptoms as dizziness, agitation, restlessness, repeated headaches, and trouble in sleeping. And in each case, the diagnosis had been anxiety neurosis until the role of caffeine was recognized.

In each case, too, symptoms disappeared when caffeine intake was cut, improvement occurring in as few as thirty-six hours.

Before making a report of his findings in the *American Journal of Psychology*, Dr. Greden did a sample check of the records of one hundred outpatients being treated for psychiatric conditions, and found that forty-two were being treated for anxiety symptoms but not one had been asked about his caffeine intake.

Individual sensitivity to caffeine varies, but for many individuals symptoms can be brought on by as little as 250 milligrams of caffeine, a dosage, Greden reports, exceeded by many people every day. For example, three cups of coffee, two headache tablets containing caffeine, and a cola drink consumed in one morning approximates 500 milligrams of caffeine intake.

Greden urges physicians to routinely question patients about caffeine intake.

(Recent studies indicate considerable variation in caffeine content per five-ounce cup of various beverages: brewed coffee, 80 to 120 milligrams; instant coffee, 66 to 100 milligrams; decaffeinated, 1 to 6 milligrams; leaf tea, 30 to 75 milligrams; bagged tea, 42 to 100 milligrams; instant tea, 30 to 60 milligrams; cocoa, up to 50 milligrams; cola drinks, 15 to 30 milligrams; chocolate bars, up to 25 milligrams.)

(EB-9)

CHAPTER 7

Eye Disorders

A new look at some old—and standing—misconceptions

Myths and misconceptions about the eyes are common and some of them lead to needless anxiety and needless, limiting inhibitions and restrictions.

A recent medical study finds that among the most common erroneous notions is the belief that eyes can be damaged either by excessive use, very fine work, or work in poor light. The facts: No such condition as eyestrain exists; straining the eyes by overuse appears to be about as impossible as straining the nose by too much smelling. Eye muscles can and do become fatigued as can muscles elsewhere in the body; and, as elsewhere, rest relieves the fatigue.

Nor are several other common notions valid: that the wearing of eyeglasses weakens the eyes or changes their condition; that the eyes can be damaged by use of sunglasses, holding reading matter too close, or watching television while seated on the floor.

Among the erroneous ideas about the eyes and sex, one of the most common is that "too much" sexual activity must impair vision. Another also common: People who squint are better lovers.   (E-1)

Bloodshot eyes from swimming: relieving and preventing them

After swimming in chlorinated pools, many people find their eyes bloodshot, and, not uncommonly, many experience burning and tearing for several hours after a swim.

But even though chlorinated water, and sometimes fresh unchlorinated water, may inflame the eyes, no instance of permanent eye damage has ever been reported, even among professional swimmers who, in addition to competing frequently, often practice many hours a day.

Suggests one physician, a member of the American Medical Association Committee on the Medical Aspects of Sports: a few drops of methylcellulose into the eyes is often valuable for relieving irritation and even as a preventive agent to help reduce irritation to a minimum.   (E-2)

"Lazy eye" (amblyopia): new developments

When a child has eyes that deviate, he may see double images. That can also happen when one eye is normal and the other is either nearsighted or farsighted, or when one eye is nearsighted and the other is farsighted. In order to stop seeing double, the brain shuts out one eye, and since that eye is not used, vision in it deteriorates.

Even when sight in one eye has deteriorated markedly, there is a good chance it can be restored. Treatment for lazy eye, when carried out early enough, can be effective. Eyeglasses and a patch over the good eye may be needed. The patch forces the use of the weak eye so that, with increased use, vision in it builds up.

A major problem, a recent study shows, is that although as many as 2 percent of children have amblyopia, in only about half of them is any eye deviation obvious; in the others, the eyes appear to be normal.

Early detection is essential. The later treatment is begun, the less the likelihood for improvement. Urges Dr. Roger L. Hiatt of the University of Tennessee, Memphis, who carried out the study: Even when a child is only a year old, if there is any suspicion that the two eyes are not seeing equally well—and at any age, even as early as three months, if one eye seems to deviate from the other—a medical examination should be performed.

Where, before age four, most amblyopic eyes can be improved with treatment, fewer become correctable between ages four and seven, still fewer after age seven.

Because of a common idea that urgently needs to be replaced—that a child's eyes need not be examined until school age—many children are being deprived of binocular vision with two eyes functioning as a team to provide true depth perception.   (E-3)

A recent development that promises to be helpful for some children with lazy eye is the use of a soft contact lens placed on the normal eye. The invisible contact lens can blur vision in the good eye enough to compel the lazy eye to begin to work and see better. It takes the place of an external eye patch, eliminating any possible adhesive irritation and averting teasing from other youngsters, sometimes a problem.

After experience with several dozen children using the contact lens, physicians at the Department of Pediatric Ophthalmology of Wills Eye Hospital, Philadelphia, report that it is "extremely advantageous" because no one notices the lens and it becomes an invisible eye patch.   (E-4)

Herpetic keratitis: an important added aid

A serious problem, herpetic keratitis is a superficial ulceration of the clear cornea covering of the eye. Its cause is the same herpes simplex virus responsible for cold sores and fever blisters. Early symptoms are foreign-body sensation, excessive tearing of the eye, excessive sensitivity to light. Left untreated, the disease may lead to permanent scarring of the cornea.

One drug, idoxuridine, helps some patients. If it fails after three to five days, the entire corneal "skin" may be removed with a sharp knife under topical anesthesia, followed by a tightly applied double patch for two to three days. Alternatively, chemical removal of the skin is sometimes used, and consists of applying to the ulcer and a wide area around it 2 percent iodine tincture, ether, or other chemicals, to remove the diseased corneal surface.

A new drug, vidarabine ointment, has been found to benefit a high proportion of patients who cannot be helped with idoxuridine. In studies by Dr. Deborah Pavan-Langston of Harvard Medical School, Boston, 87 percent of more than one hundred patients not benefited by idoxuridine have responded to vidarabine.   (E-5)

New hope for keratoconus

In keratoconus, an abnormal conical protrusion of the central part of the cornea results in irregular astigmatism, and may seriously interfere with vision.

At the University of Florida School of Medicine, a research team headed by Dr. Antonio Gasset has developed a treatment for keratoconus which, in early clinical trial, has shown promise.

Called thermokeratoplasty, it involves quick and gentle heating of the cornea by application of a small heating probe. The procedure takes no more than a minute. Over a period of several months afterward, the cornea flattens so the conical protrusion gradually disappears.

In the first ten patients, Dr. Gasset has reported, vision has improved from that of legal blindness (20/200 or less vision in one or both eyes) to at least 20/40 and in some cases to 20/20.   (E-6)

Restoring vision to eyes blinded by vitreous hemorrhage

Less than half a dozen years ago, blindness caused by vitreous hemorrhage—escape of blood from a vessel into the vitreous humor, the transparent substance filling the part of the eyeball between the lens and the retina—was beyond hope. Now, in many cases, it is no longer so.

Vitreous hemorrhage may occur as the result of diabetes or rupture of a retinal vessel because of disease or injury. Sometimes the blood is absorbed spontaneously and fairly rapidly. But if spontaneous absorption does not occur, no medical treatment has promoted absorption of the blood, which then obscures vision and, in time in some cases, may lead to detachment of the retina.

Now a new operation, called a vitrectomy, uses a new surgical instrument, a vitrophage, with which an ophthalmologist can cut open the eye, suck out the clouded vitreous, temporarily instill a saline solution to maintain internal eye pressure, and finally reinfuse the vitreous after the blood has been removed. Then the jellylike mass once again is a clear medium for transmitting light between the lens and the retina.

One of the first to develop the technique, Dr. Nicholas Douvas of Port Huron, Michigan, has reported that out of the first twenty-five patients operated on, all selected to make certain their retinas were still functioning and not detached, only seven have failed to achieve sight. Among the patients is one man blind for five years who now has 20/40 vision; another was blind for two years but now is able to read tiny want-ad print.

At the University of Illinois in Chicago, Dr. Gholam Peyman, who independently developed a slightly different form of the instrument, has reported restoration of useful vision in ten of some twenty blind and near-blind patients.

The operation takes three hours. It is done under a microscope. Patients may be kept in the hospital at least a week. The operation is not risk-free since it requires working within the eyeball. Thus there is always a chance—"slim but real," Dr. Peyman calls it—of injuring the retina. However, when the operation is used for blind eyes, patients, as Dr. Douvas puts it, "have nothing to lose and everything to gain." (E-7)

Relieving uncontrollable eyelid twitching

In a condition called essential blepharospasm, the eyelids contract uncontrollably. The cause is unknown. Both eyes are usually involved, and vision is impaired by the eye-closing spasms, which often become progressively more severe and long-lasting.

Surgery to remove segments of facial nerve, according to Drs. Brian F. McCabe of the University of Iowa, Iowa City, and Roger Boles of the University of Michigan Medical Center, Ann Arbor, is often effective for bringing the spasms under control, and in their experience over a number of years the satisfactory results persist. (E-8)

Glaucoma: New aids to control

Its cause unknown, glaucoma is characterized by abnormal elevation of pressure within the eye and impaired vision.

Commonly, side vision is lost first and the patient in effect seems to be looking down a rifle barrel. There may also be fogged vision and appearance of colored rings around bright objects. When uncontrolled, central vision is lost.

For many of the almost two million people in the United States who have glaucoma, a new way to take medication, in the form of a tiny oval wafer tipped into the eye once a week, could be helpful.

Although drugs have been available to control most cases of glaucoma, the disease nevertheless is responsible for about 12 percent of all cases of adult blindness. And many studies have indicated that much of the problem may lie with poor patient compliance. At several glaucoma clinics where the problem has been studied, more than half the patients have been found to use eyedrops improperly or fail to use them at all.

The drops must be instilled at frequent intervals, which discourages some patients. Getting them into the eyes is sometimes a hit-and-miss proposition. Some patients may be discouraged, too, by the fact that blurring of vision for an hour or so may occur after instillation.

The new wafer, called Ocusert, recently released by the United States Food and Drug Administration for prescription by ophthalmologists, is designed to overcome many of these difficulties.

It represents a considerable triumph of technology. The tiny wafer—only ¼ inch by ½ inch by 1/10 inch thick—placed in the eye once a week and left there releases one of the most reliable drugs, pilocarpine, at a uniform rate over the week, usually without blurring or other unpleasant effects.

At a casual glance, the wafer appears to be a simple, flexible film. Actually, it is a multicomponent precision system. A central reservoir of drug is sandwiched between two special and remarkable membranes that permit controlled release of the medication.

The little wafer—which, because of the uniform controlled release, needs to contain only about one-eighth of the amount of drug usually required in eyedrop form four times a day—is easily picked up on a clean fingertip and placed under the lower eyelid. Once in place, it is invisible and does not restrict normal activities, including swimming.

Reports from investigators at many medical centers indicate that the wafer system—which works on the premise that low doses of pilocarpine, if administered continuously, can control intraocular pressure—does in fact produce pressure reduction with minimal disturbances of visual acuity and minimal other adverse reactions.

Not all patients like it. Some 18 percent dropped out of studies for one reason or other. But the majority of patients have had little or no difficulty with the wafers and consider them advantageous. Many who used to find every drop instillation an ordeal are enthusiastic, finding the once-a-week wafer placement simple, and their adaptability to its presence is so high that they are unaware of it throughout the week.

A main problem is price—about seven times greater than for drops. The cost stems from the intricate technology; the tiny wafer components must have tolerances of as little as 0.0005 inch, and much of the manufacturing operation is carried out by hand under magnification.

The same technology is being studied for application to other important problems, including possibly more effective administration of antiviral drugs for serious virus-related eye diseases.   (E-9)

Not all patients, however, have glaucoma amenable to treatment with the usual medications. For at least some of them, a drug, 6-hydroxydopamine (6HD) may hold promise.

At Tulane University School of Medicine, Dr. Monte G. Holland has reported on using the drug in treating 128 eyes of ninety-two glaucomatous patients, in most of whom intraocular pressure could not be controlled with previous medical treatment and, in some cases, surgical treatment.

The drug so increased many patient's responsiveness to epinephrine, another medication often used for glaucoma control, that in 65 percent who had previously failed to respond to treatment, an average 83 percent greater reduction in intraocular pressure was achieved, bringing the glaucoma under effective control.   (E-10)

CHAPTER 8

Gastrointestinal Disorders

Chronic heartburn: new insights, new treatment

Except for the common cold, there may be nothing as commonly discomforting for so many people as what physicians call "symptomatic gastroesophageal reflux" and victims know better as "heartburn."

In heartburn, with its burning pain along the course of the esophagus, or gullet, some of the stomach contents leak back upward into the esophagus. Since acid is present in those contents (it is harmless in the stomach, which is normally protected against it, but is irritating in the esophagus, which lacks such protection), the heartburn symptom occurs.

Relief from antacids is transient, lasting only as long as they are able to continue to neutralize the acid—at best, about forty-five minutes.

If antacids may be helpful insofar as they provide fleeting relief— and some people with chronic heartburn take them hourly—they do nothing for the cause.

Recent studies at the United States Naval Hospital at Philadelphia and elsewhere have determined what the basic mechanism in chronic heartburn usually is and have opened a new approach to treatment.

Where the esophagus or gullet leads into the stomach, there is a circular, purse-string kind of muscle, a sphincter, sometimes referred to as the lower esophageal sphincter (LES). Its job is to open to permit food to pass into the stomach, then close to prevent any return (reflux) of stomach contents back up into the esophagus.

The studies have shown that heartburn occurs when the sphincter pressure is inadequate. With low sphincter pressure there is less of a barrier against reflux. Almost ten years ago, studies began to establish that patients with chronic heartburn have decreased LES pressures as compared with normal persons.

More recently, at the Philadelphia hospital, a team of gastroenterologists—Commanders Raymond L. Farrell and Gerald T. Roling and Captain Donald O. Castell—began to study agents that might possibly increase LES pressure and thus might provide a new approach to treating patients with refractory heartburn.

A promising drug proved to be bethanechol, previously used in patients suffering from urinary retention and abdominal distention after surgery.

In a first study, the navy physicians used bethanechol in eleven chronic heartburn sufferers, all longtime, heavy users of the many antacids on the market, and in eleven normal persons.

With a catheter (tubelike) device placed in the esophagus, the doctors could measure sphincter pressure continuously. After a fifteen-minute base period, the drug was injected subcutaneously and pressures were measured for another hour.

In the normal persons, the mean base pressure was 14.6 milligrams of mercury; after the injection it peaked to 31.5. In the chronic heartburn patients, the mean basal pressure of 4.31 rose to a peak of 19.6.

Then the chronic heartburn patients were given twenty-five milligrams of bethanechol by mouth and their pressures were measured for two hours. They rose to a peak of 16.9 and remained elevated throughout the two hours.

More recently, the navy physicians carried out a scientifically controlled trial with twenty patients with chronic heartburn poorly controlled by antacids. The group consisted of fourteen men and six women, ranging in age from twenty-five to seventy-five, suffering with chronic heartburn from two to twenty years.

Each patient received bethanechol tablets for two months and identical-appearing inert tablets for two months, with neither physicians nor patients knowing who was receiving what until the trial was over and the medication code was broken.

The results of the trial were clearcut: 25-milligram bethanechol tablets four times a day decreased heartburn symptoms and antacid consumption in the twenty patients who previously had suffered with heartburn despite continued antacid use.   (GI-1)

Smoking and heartburn. That smoking is often a factor in heartburn has been demonstrated by British investigators.

At the Royal Infirmary in Hull, England, Drs. C. Stanciu and J. R. Bennett studied a group of twenty-five volunteers—sixteen men and nine women, aged twenty-four to seventy-one, all chronic smokers and heartburn sufferers.

Measuring devices were used to record esophageal sphincter pressures. Pressures fell by a mean of about 40 percent during smoking, beginning within one to four minutes after a cigarette was lighted. It climbed back up three to eight minutes after the cigarette was finished.

The measuring devices also permitted recording of any increase in acidity in the esophagus as an indication that reflux of acid from the stomach was taking place. During a fifteen-hour period, for the twenty-five patients as a whole, 226 refluxes occurred, seventy-one of them during smoking, and twenty-six within eight minutes after a cigarette was finished (129 were unconnected with smoking). Heartburn occurred with 68 percent of the refluxes experienced while smoking, with 65 percent of those happening after smoking, and with 56 percent of the nonsmoking episodes.   (GI-2)

A hard new look at the value (if any) of diets for gastrointestinal disorders

What should the patient with a common gastrointestinal disorder eat?

Even in the early sixties, a detailed report by the American Medical Association's Council on Foods and Nutrition pointed out that diet treatment for most digestive tract problems was based on unsubstantiated opinion and tradition.

Much more recently, another report pointed out that, with a few very specific exceptions, the situation remained as muddled as ever.

A prime example of the muddle: dietary treatment of peptic ulcer.

Observed the latest report by Dr. Robert M. Donaldson of Boston University School of Medicine: "Those who advocate dietary restrictions for ulcer patients urge that only 'bland' foods be allowed. In general that restriction has been implemented by presenting the patient with foods of a particular color (white), consistency (soft), and taste (mild) that fits the physician's or dietitian's preconceived notion of what is bland. It is clear, however, that what is considered bland in one set of dietary instructions may be different from what is permissible in another.

"There is something fundamentally wrong with an approach that assumes that the form, consistency, color, taste and odor of a food have anything to do with the effects of that food on secretions, mucosal integrity, vascularity or motility of the gastrointestinal tract. Controlled clinical trials indicate that the kinds of food ingested have no effect on the course of peptic disease or on the quantity of acid in the stomach."

There seems to be little doubt, the report concluded, that the ulcer patient should be allowed after all to enjoy his food.

Similar confusion exists for other gastrointestinal disorders, such as biliary tract disease (gallbladder), regional enteritis, ulcerative colitis, diverticulitis, and functional bowel disorders. Except that withdrawal of milk may benefit some, but by no means all, patients with ulcerative colitis, there is no satisfactory evidence that what the patient eats affects any of these disorders, the report noted.

What if you decide that in your personal experience a particular food causes stomach trouble for you? Don't eat it, advises the report, but at the same time don't assume that just because it seems to bother you it will necessarily be bad for someone else with a similar condition.

With a few exceptions, such as eliminating certain sugars in patients with known defects in sugar digestion, and eliminating coffee and alcohol in active ulcer patients, "there seems to be little need for the patient with gastrointestinal disease and his physician to become entangled in confusing dicta about what to eat," the report indicated.   (GI-3)

Dietary fiber and bowel disorders

An increasing amount of evidence indicates that lack of fiber in the diet may contribute significantly to the development of many bowel disorders, and that restoration of fiber often may help to control those disorders.

Until about the turn of the century, man ate much fiber. It is the indigestible part of plant cell walls, present naturally in large amounts in grains and cereals.

With the invention late in the 1800s of the modern roller mill, it became economically feasible to remove the outer husk of cereal grain kernels, and with it the fiber, to produce refined white flour. Today, fiber intake in the United States is one-tenth of what it once was.

As fiber intake has gone down, the incidence of many bowel disorders has gone up. Appendicitis, for example, became common only in this century. Cancer of the colon has become, after lung cancer, the second most common cause of cancer death. Diverticular disease—abnormal outpouchings of the colon that can cause severe discomfort and may require surgery to remove the affected section of the bowel—affects one-third of Americans over age forty. Constipation is a widespread problem. So, too, is the irritable bowel syndrome—also called spastic colon and mucous colitis—with abdominal distention, cramps or dull deep pain, belching, nausea, weakness, faintness, and headaches.

But even as these disorders have been increasing in the United States and other Western nations, investigators have discovered, they remain rare among rural Africans living on native unrefined diets, containing large amounts of fiber.

It has become evident, too, that as Africans move from villages to cities and adopt Western diets with refined foods, the incidence of all the bowel disorders climbs rapidly.

Moreover, a striking change in incidence has occurred among American blacks whose ancestors came from African villages where even today colon cancer, for example, is rare. Even fifty years ago, when black and white American menus differed substantially, bowel cancer affected two whites for every black. Now, with diets virtually the same, blacks are affected as often as whites.

The mechanism. Fibrous foods add bulk. The fiber, once in the gastrointestinal tract, absorbs water and swells. That makes stools soft and large, preventing constipation with its small, hard, pebbly, slow-moving stools. Native African stools weigh four times those of westerners, and transit time—the interval from eating a meal until the remains are evacuated—averages only thirty-five hours for African villagers, ninety hours for many westerners.

More than a nuisance in itself, constipation—a rarity in rural Africans, extremely common here—leads to straining at stool, which can set the stage for a series of disorders.

With straining, it has been shown, pressure in the colon is raised and pushes on the colon wall, leading to the outpouchings of diverticular disease. Also, with straining, pressure within the abdomen is increased and may, some investigators believe, tend to raise the stomach up through the diaphragm, causing hiatal hernia, a condition that sometimes leads to heartburn and other discomfort.

(In the opinion of some investigating physicians now, raised intraabdominal pressure can be transmitted to the leg veins, dilating them to produce varicose veins, and to veins in the anal area, dilating them to produce hemorrhoids, which are, in fact, varicose veins.)

As for cancer of the colon, there is evidence that cancer-causing (carcinogenic) chemicals produced by bacteria in the bowel are involved. With the small, hard, slow-moving stools of constipation, colon cancer may be promoted in two ways: by giving the bacteria more time to act on the stools and produce carcinogens and also by giving the carcinogens more time to act on the colon lining.

Corrective effects. Many recent British studies at the Royal Infirmary, Bristol, indicate that restoring fiber to the diet has clearly measurable corrective value.

In one study with both adults and children, the use of just two slices of fiber-rich whole-meal bread in place of the same amount of white bread and the addition of two teaspoonsful (about one half ounce) of fiber-rich bran a day produced within three weeks marked increases in stool weights and speedup of transit time, ending constipation.

Until very recently, so-called "roughage" was a medical taboo for patients with diverticular disease. Now physicians have become aware that restoring dietary fiber often helps patients with the disease. In one British study, 88.6 percent of patients improved, including many who had been scheduled for, but no longer required, surgery.

Irritable colon has responded to a high-fiber diet in British studies and more recently in a study by Dr. J. L. Piepmeyer of the Beaufort,

North Carolina, Naval Hospital in which improvement occurred in 88 percent of patients.

Meanwhile, long-term studies of the possible value of dietary fiber in other gastrointestinal conditions are under way.

Restoring the fiber. Certain breakfast cereals such as old-fashioned, slow-cooking (not "instant") oatmeal, shredded wheat, and whole-grain wheat cereals are fiber-rich. Cereals with "bran" in their name contain sizeable amounts of fiber.

Whole-meal breads and whole-meal flour are rich in fiber, and the flour can be substituted in many recipes calling for white flour, including those for making your own bread, rolls, muffins, and pancakes.

Many vegetables and fruit—particularly mango, carrot, apple, Brussels sprout, eggplant, cabbage, orange, pear, green beans, lettuce, peas, onion, celery, cucumber, broad beans, tomato, cauliflower, banana, rhubarb, potato, and turnip contain dietary fiber.

Unprocessed bran—discarded in the milling of white flour—is available in health-food stores and may be in others. It can be used, not as a replacement for other sources of dietary fiber, but as a supplement, sprinkled on cereals, mixed with soup, and combined with flour in baking.   (GI-4)

Healing chronic stomach ulcers

Glycopyrronium bromide—a drug that controls excess stomach acidity and excess stomach motility—appears to be a useful agent for chronic stomach ulcers.

In a comparison study at the University of Sydney, Australia, one group of patients received such conventional treatment as bed rest and antacids as needed while another group received the same treatment plus glycopyrronium bromide.

Initial healing was accelerated in those receiving the drug, and its regular use after healing, the investigators also report, seems to protect against recurrence and has done so in patients followed for as long as four years.   (GI-5)

Ulcer and other gastrointestinal bleeding

Surgery often has been needed to control bleeding peptic ulcers and other gastrointestinal lesions.

In many cases, surgery may be avoided by a procedure recently reported to the American College of Gastroenterology by Dr. John P. Papp of Grand Rapids, Michigan.

An endoscope—a lighted tube—is passed through the throat into the stomach to locate the bleeding site and immediately, through the endoscope, a second instrument is passed to coagulate the bleeding area electrically.

Of nine patients with duodenal ulcers, only two experienced bleeding again after coagulation. Of nine with stomach ulcers, only two re-bled and needed surgery.

Patients with gastritis and other hemorrhaging lesions also have been successfully treated thus, Dr. Papp has reported, with shortening of hospitalization and substantial savings.   (GI-6)

Another new medical method is showing promise for massive hemorrhage from stress ulcer—a stomach or duodenal ulcer that characteristically bleeds very heavily under stress, after surgery, or following use of cortisone.

Although medical treatment frequently has been ineffective and even surgery has failed to save life in some cases, 75 percent of a group of patients have responded to doses of human growth hormone. Bleeding has been controlled and healing has followed, report Dr. Sidney J. Winawer and a team of physicians of Memorial Sloan-Kettering Cancer Center and Cornell University Medical College, New York City.   (GI-7)

Diarrhea: new developments

To treat or not to treat. Is a short bout of diarrhea harmful? On the contrary, if unpleasant, it may nevertheless be beneficial, nature's method of hastening out of the gastrointestinal tract disease-producing agents before they do much damage. And a rush to use medication to stop such diarrhea without delay may cause increased illness.

So report physicians of the University of Texas Medical School, Houston, and the University of Maryland School of Medicine, Baltimore, after a study with twenty-five volunteers deliberately made ill with infectious diarrhea.

Some were given a drug (Lomotil) often prescribed for diarrhea control. Their diarrhea was, indeed, controlled sooner but they had fever much longer than others not receiving the drug.   (GI-8)

Giardia lamblia diarrhea. One of the major causes—and a frequently unrecognized one—of gastrointestinal upsets among travelers is a parasite, Giardia lamblia. Prevalent in warm climates, especially in the feces of children, it is passed on in the form of a cyst which can produce cramps, nausea, mucous diarrhea, fatigue, and appetite and weight loss.

One effective drug is the antimalarial, quinacrine hydrochloride, which can eradicate the parasite and the symptoms. In a study at the Palo Alto Medical Clinic, Palo Alto, California, all of seventy patients responded to 100-milligram doses of quinacrine hydrochloride taken three or four times a day.   (GI-9)

Fiber for diarrhea. Although whole-meal breads, bran, and other high-fiber foods are known to be good for constipation, conventionally they have been banned for diarrhea.

Yet, in some cases, it now appears, patients who have nonspecific diarrhea—not related to any infectious process or other disease—may benefit from a high-fiber intake.

At the University of Bristol, England, investigators studied twenty volunteers who for four weeks switched from their usual refined diet to one high in fiber.

As expected, among those in the group with a tendency to constipation, intestinal transit time was speeded up by the high-fiber intake. Unexpectedly, in those with a tendency to diarrhea, the transit time slowed, minimizing the diarrhea.   (GI-10)

A resin for unyielding diarrhea of unknown cause. Cholestyramine, a resin taken in powder form, has been used to lower blood cholesterol levels. Now it has been reported to benefit, often dramatically, patients suffering from intractable diarrhea of unknown cause, although how it does so is unknown.

At Massachusetts General Hospital, when cholestyramine was given for four days to patients with diarrhea that had resisted treatment for months or years, 50 percent responded quickly and dramatically. After using eight grams a day to stop the diarrhea, Dr. Robert H. Shapiro of the hospital has found, a maintenance dose of two grams a day is satisfactory. About half of patients have a recurrence if the maintenance dose is stopped.

At the University of Miami School of Medicine, Dr. M. A. Tamer and other pediatricians resorted to cholestyramine for a group of infants, aged two to twenty-four weeks, with diarrhea lasting ten to twenty-five days, cause unknown. They were resistant to treatment that had included three antibiotics, intravenous fluid replacement, and special formulates. The diarrhea was eliminated with four to eight grams a day of cholestyramine for six days and the diarrhea did not recur after the drug was stopped.   (GI-11)

Hiatal hernia: some strange effects

Hiatal or hiatus hernia (both terms are used) is a peculiar problem. Any hernia is a rupture that permits an organ to protrude through. The esophagus, or gullet, passes through the diaphragm, the strong, dome-shaped muscle that separates chest from abdominal cavity. In hiatal hernia, part of the stomach pushes up through the opening in the diaphragm where the esophagus passes through, entering the chest cavity, either intermittently or constantly.

Often the hernia produces no symptoms at all. When the condition is symptomatic, the most common symptoms are heartburn, regurgitation of gastric juices from the stomach to the esophagus, and burning pain behind the breastbone. The pain, which is worse after eating and when lifting or stooping, sometimes may resemble the anginal chest pain associated with heart disease.

Hiatal hernia, when suspected, can be diagnosed with the help of X-rays taken after a swallow of barium, a contrast material that helps to show up the herniation. In some cases, surgery may be needed, but very often medical treatment that may include such simple measures as elevation of the head of the bed for sleep and use of antacids is satisfactory.

But hiatal hernia apparently sometimes can produce confusing symptoms—sensations of a foreign body caught in the throat, hoarseness, neck pain, earache, or stubborn cough—which may occur without any of the usual hiatal hernia symptoms.

The strange symptoms occurred in a group of twenty-two patients seen by two Washington, D.C., physicians, Drs. J. D. Hallewell and T. B. Cole. In twenty-one, the usual medical measures for hiatal hernia provided relief; one patient required surgery.   (GI-12)

The stomach "lump" that isn't

What may seem to be a suspicious lump in the stomach worries many people—needlessly. In his experience, one physician has reported, the worriers most often are young men, who vacillate for months before seeking medical advice as they become increasingly anxious over the possibility that it is a malignant growth.

Yet a medical check quickly shows that the seeming lump is really a normal xiphoid process, a point of bone and cartilage connected with the lower end of the breastbone.   (GI-13)

Milk intolerance

Abdominal bloating, unexplained abdominal cramps, or diarrhea can be the results in some cases of an intolerance for milk.

Commonly, people with the intolerance are otherwise healthy and drank milk without ill effects as children.

Their intolerance has nothing to do with allergy but rather involves a deficiency of an intestinal enzyme needed for digesting the lactose constituent of milk.

In a study by Dr. Theodore M. Bayless of Johns Hopkins University School of Medicine, Baltimore, people with milk intolerance because of the enzyme deficiency, unable to handle large amounts of milk, often could take smaller amounts in cereals and coffee and also had less difficulty if they took milk with their meals rather than alone.

Ice-cold milk especially is to be avoided, Bayless has found. He has also found that the intolerant usually do well with forms of milk such as yogurt and cheese in which part of the lactose has been converted to another substance.   (GI-14)

A treatment for taste disturbances

Taste disturbances—loss of all taste or distortions that make normal foods taste foul—have often been considered to be psychological in origin.

Recently, however, they have been traced in many cases to a deficiency of the metal zinc, which is required by the body in small amounts.

Dr. Robert I. Henkin of the National Heart and Lung Institute, Bethesda, Maryland, has reported a study of 103 patients with taste disturbances. They ranged in age from twenty-five to eighty-one years and were found to have abnormally low levels of zinc in their blood.

When given zinc sulfate in doses of 25, 50, or 100 milligrams four times a day, all showed increases in zinc blood levels, about two-thirds regained normal taste, and the remainder experienced marked improvement.   (GI-15)

To stop choking on food

Choking on a piece of food, very often a large chunk of meat, is a much more common problem than generally realized and can be fatal. Many so-called "café coronaries," sudden deaths in restaurants which have seemed to be the result of heart attacks, were in reality the result of choking on food.

If you should ever experience such choking, urges Dr. Theodore H. Ingalls of Framingham, Massachusetts, summon all the air in your lungs for one vigorous cough. Cough immediately, without leaving the table; there isn't time enough to get to a rest room. "When you are stoppered like a bottle with a cork in it, you must hack with whatever remaining air you can squeeze from your lungs," he advises. (GI-16)

A "hug of life" maneuver to be used when you see a dinner partner suddenly choking on food has been developed by Dr. Henry Heimlich of the Jewish Hospital, Cincinnati, and has been endorsed by both the American Medical Association and the American Red Cross.

To carry it out, stand in back of the victim, reach both your arms around him, make a fist, and grasp the fist with the other hand. Then, placing the thumb side of the fist against the victim's abdomen above the navel but below the rib cage, press your fist sharply upward. This raises the diaphragm, compresses the lungs, and increases the air pressure in the windpipe, forcing the food particle out. In an eighteen-month period, the hug of life used on some 374 potential victims, including one nine months old, led to survival for all.

CHAPTER 9

Genitourinary Disorders

A vitamin for a puzzling urethritis

Urethritis, an inflammation of the urethra, the canal extending from the bladder and opening to the outside of the body, may cause both increased urination and urgency to urinate, along with burning pain on urination and sometimes a purulent discharge.

It frequently is a symptom of gonorrhea or another infection and antibiotic treatment then usually works. But in some men no infection can be found, and in at least some of these mysterious cases, Dr. Stephen N. Rous of the New York Medical College-Metropolitan Hospital Center has determined, the problem may lie with a persistently alkaline, irritative urine, and vitamin C may be helpful.

When urine becomes strongly alkaline, it no longer can hold in solution, as it normally does, phosphate crystals, which then, like cinders in the eye, produce discomfort.

This appeared to be the trouble in a group of a dozen men. All responded to massive doses of vitamin C (ascorbic acid)—3 grams a day for four days—which acidified the urine, permitting it to dissolve the irritating crystals.   (GU-1)

The most common—and unrecognized and untreated—venereal disease?

Gonorrhea has long been considered the most common venereal disease in the United States, but a more common cause of genital infection, some recent studies suggest, may be the same organism, Chlamydia trachomatis, that, when it invades the eye, causes trachoma.

In one study among male college students, evidence suggested that as much as 92 percent of urethritis was nongonococcal and that at least half of the nongonococcal cases were associated with chlamydial infection.

While gonococcal infection appears to be more common among lower socioeconomic groups, chlamydial infection appears to be more common in higher socioeconomic groups.

What often happens in the case of chlamydial urethritis, according to Dr. King K. Holmes of the University of Washington, is that a physician may simply reassure the patient that it is not gonorrhea, or may treat the patient with antibiotics. Since it is not gonococcal, he will make no attempt to find and treat the patient's sexual contacts, so allowing a reservoir of infection to persist in women who may have no symptoms.

Once thought to be viruses, chlamydia organisms more recently have been found to have some characteristics similar to those of bacteria and are now considered to be "intermediate agents." They respond to antibacterial drugs, of which the most effective appear to be tetracycline and sulfa compounds.

Only recently have complex testing procedures for identifying chlamydia been developed. They still are not available to most physicians.

But Dr. Holmes and his University of Washington associates have been treating nongonococcal urethritis patients with two grams of tetracycline hydrochloride a day for seven days and finding the treatment effective for 80 percent of those among them with chlamydial infection. They have recommended that all nongonococcal patients and their sex partners, many of whom are likely to have chlamydia, be treated with tetracycline.   (GU-2)

A promising preventive for calcium kidney stone formers

Not all kidney stones are painful; some are silent. But on occasion, they may cause agonizing pain.

Calcium kidney stones are a common type and in patients who are chronic formers a low-calcium diet, avoiding all dairy products and egg yolk, may be used.

A hopeful new development is the finding that allopurinol, a drug often used for gout patients, may help minimize calcium stone formation.

In gout, uric acid, a normal body chemical, is produced in excessive amounts and accumulates painfully in joints. In studying calcium kidney stone formers, Dr. Frederic L. Coe of Michael Reese Medical Center, Chicago, found that they often have high levels of uric acid even though they have no gout symptoms.

Allopurinol is effective for gout because it interferes with body production of uric acid. On the theory that excess uric acid, even when it produces no gout, may be related to calcium stone formation, Dr. Coe tried allopurinol in twenty-one patients who had formed a total of seventy-three stones. On allopurinol over a two-year period, twenty formed no stones at all and one formed only a single stone.   (GU-3)

The prostate: benign enlargement and cancer

Benign prostatic hypertrophy—nonmalignant enlargement of the prostate gland—is common, particularly in men over sixty. Its cause is unknown. In some cases, the enlargement may be great enough to obstruct the bladder outlet and produce such symptoms as urinary frequency and urgency because of incomplete emptying of the bladder. When necessary, surgery to remove the prostate produces relief.

Understandably, many men with benign hypertrophy and even some physicians have worried over the possibility that the enlargement may increase the risk of developing cancer of the prostate.

The results of a recent study are reassuring.

New York State Department of Health investigators followed for more than ten years a group of 838 men with enlargement and another group of 802 men, matched for age, without enlargement.

In the ten-year period, twenty-four of the men with enlargement and twenty-five of the others developed prostate cancer, indicating no increased risk of cancer associated with enlargement.   (GU-4)

Zinc for prostate disorders

Zinc is one of a class of substances known as trace minerals present in the body in only the tiniest amounts and as little understood today as were vitamins seventy-five years ago. Some are known to have vital functions—iodine, for example, is required for thyroid gland functioning. Others are suspected to be no less important.

Recent studies have indicated that zinc may accelerate wound healing, that it may be needed for growth, and that a deficiency of it may produce taste and smell disturbances.

Recently, too, the work of Dr. Irving M. Bush at Cook County Hospital, Chicago, suggests that zinc deficiency may be related to some prostate gland disorders.

Although zinc is present in all body tissues in trace amounts, the prostate gland appears to have particular need for relatively large amounts and normally has one of the highest concentrations.

With the idea that low concentrations of zinc might be involved in some prostate problems, Dr. Bush studied the effect of using 50 to 150 milligrams a day of zinc sulfate as a diet supplement in two hundred men with chronic abacterial prostatitis (nonbacterial inflammation of the gland). In 70 percent, he has reported, urinary frequency, irritation, and other symptoms were relieved.

Bush has also reported trying the same treatment in a group of men with benign prostatic hypertrophy and noting reduction in the size of the gland in almost three of every four.   (GU-5)

New aids for organic impotence

Impotence—inability to attain or sustain an erection satisfactory for normal intercourse—has many possible causes. Among them are systemic diseases such as diabetes, inflammatory diseases of the genitalia, and, commonly, psychic factors. Suitable treatment for such problems often overcomes impotence.

For some years, for organic impotence not amenable to treatment with usual methods, rigid implantable penile devices have been of some help, although not really satisfactory.

Recently, two new devices have been reported in early trials to be more promising for men with impotence due to injuries, neurologic or blood-vessel disease, and other organic problems.

One, developed by Dr. F. Brantley Scott, professor of urology at

Baylor College of Medicine, Houston, consists of two inflatable silicone rubber cylinders connected by tubing to a water reservoir and a bulb actuator. The cylinders are inserted through a 6-inch or smaller incision starting at the base of the penis. The small bulb actuator is implanted into the scrotum and connected by tubing to the cylinders and to a fluid reservoir.

In a first series of sixteen patients, after a six-week postoperative waiting period, thirteen have become sexually active. When intercourse is desired, the bulb is squeezed, pumping fluid into the cylinders, causing them to expand, gradually producing erection. After intercourse, a release valve on the bulb is used to end the erection.

A less complex device developed by Dr. Michael P. Small of the University of Miami School of Medicine is made of two thin silicone sponge shafts that are implanted. Although they hold the penis erect all the time, it is bendable and can be worn inconspicuously under jockey shorts. In a first series of twenty-six patients ranging in age from nineteen to seventy-five, Dr. Small has reported, twenty-three have been able to resume sexual activity, usually within two to three weeks. The device is so simple that most urologists can install it successfully, according to Dr. Small.   (GU-6)

Controlling previously uncontrollable urinary incontinence

Previously intractable urinary incontinence in men, women, and children, resulting from neurologic disease, stress, prostate surgery, or other causes, may be controlled now in many cases by an implantable prosthetic device.

The prosthesis consists of an inflatable cuff that encircles the urethra (the canal carrying urine from bladder to outside), plus a pumping mechanism connected by internal tubing to two external small bulbs, one on each side of the scrotum or labia.

By squeezing one bulb, the patient can pump up the cuff which then remains inflated, serving to contain urine, until, at some desired time, the patient squeezes the other bulb to deflate the cuff and allow urine to flow.

Most of the first patients—thirty-four men, women, and children ranging in age from three years to seventy-six—for whom the prosthesis has been used have become continent, report Drs. F. Brantley Scott and William E. Bradley of Baylor College of Medicine, Houston, and G. W. Timm of the University of Minnesota.   (GU-7)

For kidney patients: new dialysis developments

Each year, some fifteen thousand Americans—men, women, and children of all ages—whose kidneys have shut down in complete failure join the thousands of others for whom regular hookup to an artificial kidney for thorough cleansing of the blood means the difference between life and death.

Human kidneys have as a main purpose the removal from the blood of waste products that would be poisonous if allowed to accumulate. No one can survive long if the cleansing action of the kidneys ceases; death comes after convulsions, vomiting, and severe pain.

In hemodialysis, blood is carried into a machine that cleans and then returns it to the body. Usually the cleansing must be carried out several times a week for five to six hours at a time.

Once performed only in major medical centers, dialysis today, after suitable training, can be carried out at home by many patients and their families.

Not only is hospital dialysis very costly—the estimated cost runs about $23,000 per year per patient—but facilities for such treatment also are sharply limited. In some areas, hospital centers have been completely filled and new patients must go elsewhere or do without.

Home dialysis is significantly less costly (according to some estimates, about $10,000 a year). It also permits a degree of independence and sense of accomplishment, some studies have shown, not found with hospital-based dialysis.

Some patients, however, are unable to cope with home dialysis because of their physical or emotional state or home conditions, and must receive treatment at a center. For them, it appears, there is another possible alternative: an outpatient dialysis center.

In a feasibility study of home and outpatient dialysis conducted in City Hospital, Elmhurst, New York, by Dr. Martin S. Neff and other physicians associated with both the hospital and the Mount Sinai School of Medicine, patients were brought into the hospital and trained in the use of home dialysis equipment. Also, an out-of-hospital facility was set up in a renovated commercial building, selected for its convenience to public transportation and proximity to the hospital.

A report on the study tells of successful maintenance of seventy-seven patients in the home treatment program, and of another 185 patients in the out-of-hospital facility, which runs at much lower cost than the parent facility in the hospital itself.

"Hospital dialysis should be reserved," the report indicates, "for acutely ill patients requiring hospital care. Maintenance dialysis can be successfully carried out at home or in an out-of-hospital facility."   (GU-8)

Dr. Belding H. Scribner of the University of Washington School of Medicine, Seattle, one of the pioneers in dialysis, recently reported to the National Kidney Foundation that, in his experience, the goal for home dialysis could well be set at 80 percent of patients, although currently only about 20 percent are on home dialysis.

"When there's a choice," he noted, "chronic illness is always better treated at home than in an institution. The more responsibility the patient has for his welfare, the better the result. And the more informed the patient is about details of treatment, and about complications and how to avoid them, the better the adjustment."

At a practical level, too, Dr. Scribner noted, home dialysis can be carried out while the patient sleeps and thus can permit a return to work and other normal activities. In most hospitals dialysis service is provided only in daytime hours.

When patients are encouraged to undertake home dialysis, there can be more than bare survival. Many can be rehabilitated, partially or fully. In one University of Washington study of 105 patients on home dialysis, 29 percent were found to be working full time, 29 percent were functioning as housewives, 7 percent worked part time, 10 percent were looking for work, and 11 percent were in school. Only 14 percent were retired or not looking for work.

"Fully rehabilitated patients are just as productive on dialysis as they were before their kidneys failed—sometimes more productive," report Drs. Armando Lindner and Kingsbury Curtis of the University of Washington School of Medicine.   (GU-9)

An improvement in dialysis technique. A problem in long-term dialysis is the hookup of patient and machine. The process only became feasible with the development of cannulae, or small tubes, of special silicone rubber that could be implanted in a patient's arm, one tube connected to an artery, the other to a vein. With these, the patient could be "plugged in" to a machine and when not in use the two cannulae ends could be joined to form a shunt through which blood could flow in the body circulatory system in normal fashion.

But in many patients after a time blood clotted in and blocked the shunt and infections sometimes developed at the skin exit sites.

As an alternative, surgeons created an artificial internal fistula or connection by attaching the radial artery in the forearm to a nearby vein. Since this is localized it causes no disturbance of overall artery and vein blood flow. Because of the direct connection to an artery, the vein became stronger and more elastic and could be repeatedly punctured with needles, one for withdrawing blood to the machine and the other for returning it.

Still, problems remained. In some patients, blood flow rates through a fistula were inadequate. In others, veins of adequate capacity were not available.

Now bovine artery material provides a promising new alternative. It comes from carotid (neck) arteries of slaughtered cattle. After removal, an artery is soaked in an enzyme solution that dissolves away flesh, fat, and muscle, leaving a tube of collagen, or fibrous connective tissue, about drinking-straw size. Treated next by a tanning process, the material becomes strong and leatherlike.

Called a bovine arterial heterograft, the material can be implanted, under local anesthesia, under the skin usually on an upper arm or forearm and inserted as a shunt between an artery and a vein. Afterward, it is visible as a raised lump under the skin—the place where needles can be inserted for dialysis hookup.

Trials at the University of Alabama Medical Center, Birmingham, the University of Miami School of Medicine, the Los Angeles County-University of Southern California Medical Center, and other major centers show a high rate of success in patients, including many with failures of previous shunts and fistulas. Both nurses at dialysis centers and spouses who help at home with dialysis consider the bovine graft superior in terms of less difficulty in needle insertion and better blood flow.   (GU-10)

Kidney transplants

According to a recent report, the Renal Transplant Registry established in 1963 by the American College of Surgeons and National Institutes of Health has recorded 16,444 human kidney transplants performed in the United States and abroad. This is believed to represent a major share of the world total.

Of the 16,444, 14,806 were first kidney grafts, 1,488 second, 131 third, and 19 fourth and subsequent transplants. Follow-up data available on 14,479 of the recipients indicate that 6,781 (46.8 percent) are alive with a functioning graft and an additional 2,979 (20.6 percent) survive without transplant function.

Approximately 1,400 of the transplants were carried out in patients under fifteen years of age. And both in the United States and elsewhere, at ages six through fifteen, girls account for up to 58 percent of all transplants. In contrast, of recipients aged sixteen through sixty-five years, more than two-thirds are male.

In the early years, the trend was to increasing use of kidneys donated by parents and siblings. But use of cadaver kidneys has increased from 56 percent of the grafts in 1967 to 70.4 percent more recently. Sibling donors are as common as parents, with 14.4 percent of grafts from siblings and 12.7 percent from parent donors.

Rejection by the body of the recipient of the donated kidney still is the dominant cause of graft failure when that occurs. The closer the tissue match between recipient and donor, the more likely the success; registry figures suggest a possible improvement in long-term survival of 15 to 20 percent for the optimally matched as against lesser degrees of close matching.

The report shows a gradual increase in the long-term survival of first transplants of cadaveric kidneys. Up to ten years ago, the five-year survival rate was 16 percent; more recently it has moved up to 35 percent.   (GU-11)

The outlook for kidney donors

What future is in store for someone who donates a kidney for transplant? Reassuring findings come from a study by Drs. A. H. Bennett and J. H. Harrison of Harvard Medical School, Boston.

Over a nineteen-year period, only one transplant-related death occurred among three hundred donors who ranged in age from twelve to eighty years and in most cases were parents or siblings of the transplant recipients.

Life expectancy with one kidney, the study indicates, is not reduced in the absence of injury to that remaining kidney. As a precaution, donors usually are advised to avoid participation in body contact sports.

Of donors who responded to a questionnaire, 92 percent reported experiencing no change in their physical condition after transplant. Most reported no change in personal relationship to the recipient; 9 percent reported a closer personal relationship.   (GU-12)

CHAPTER 10

Geriatric Problems

Senile dementia: new help from brain scanners

It is increasingly recognized today that senile dementia in many cases has been a wastebasket diagnosis—a consignment to hopelessness. In older people there has been a strong tendency to link intellectual failings and dementia with aging brain arteries and brain atrophy without possibility of reversal.

Very recently, however, many studies have been suggesting that some of the seemingly senile elderly, even some of those with hardening of brain arteries and atrophy, have other problems that contribute to their plight—among them, anemia, mental depression, heart failure, hypertension—and that correction of these problems may bring significant improvement in personality and mental functioning even though artery hardening and brain atrophy remain.   (GE-1)

Among the particularly hopeful new developments is the beginning of use of the new brain scanning machines for diagnosis. The brain scanners use a technique called CAT (computerized axial tomography), in which information obtained with a special X-ray beam that shoots out to 160 different areas of the brain is picked up and processed by a computer which then turns out a picture. Unlike conventional X-ray devices that provide only two-dimensional pictures, the scanners provide three-dimensional ones and have the ability to reveal details and data never before available.

The scanners, for example, can reveal brain atrophy, cysts, abscesses, tumors of the brain, blood vessel malformations, and much more.

Scanning is a simple noninvasive procedure. No injections of any kind are required. With the patient lying comfortably, the scanning is carried out within a few minutes.   (GE-2)

In one of the first reports on use of brain scanning for elderly people thought to be suffering from hopeless senile dementia, a team of physicians at Rush-Presbyterian-Saint Luke's Medical Center, Chicago—Drs. M. S. Huckman, Jacob Fox, and Jordan Topel—has noted that although it has been assumed that senile dementia is present when conventional X-ray films show cerebral atrophy or diminished brain size, with the new technique some demented patients have been found to have only moderate or even questionable atrophy.

And in several such patients, when other possible problems were sought—among them, low thyroid functioning and pernicious anemia—and then vigorously treated, dementia was almost completely relieved.

As the Chicago team has noted, "This suggests that absence of major atrophy shown by CAT in a demented patient should make the physician particularly suspicious of a potentially treatable illness."

Brain scanners—and whole body scanners operating on the same principle—are in increasing use now, already installed in well over one hundred major medical centers and large hospitals and with more being installed each month.

Improving blood flow to the senile brain

Several recent studies suggest that at least in some patients with senile dementia, medical treatment to try to improve blood flow to the brain, either alone or coupled with psychotherapy, may be of value.

At Western Psychiatric Institute and Clinic, Pittsburgh, Dr. Arthur C. Walsh has used psychotherapy combined with Dicumarol, an anticoagulant drug that thins the blood and in so doing may facilitate its flow through hardened, narrowed arteries in the brain. His patients, ranging in age up to eighty-nine, have suffered from impaired judgment, memory loss, and confusion. By the end of two months, he has reported, 90 percent of the patients showed improvement. (GE-3)

In England, at Powick Hospital, Worcestershire, Dr. Peter Hall has been carrying out trials with cyclandelate, a drug that dilates blood vessels and may help to improve blood flow.

He has reported results thus far in a trial with twenty-one patients, aged to eighty-eight, who sometimes received the drug and at other times, for comparison, a look-alike but inert preparation.

During active drug treatment, improvement occurred in mental state, mood, orientation, memory, and abstraction. "Cyclandelate and perhaps other drugs—together with supportive and rehabilitative measures—offer some hope," reports Dr. Hall, "of improving the ability of these patients to cope with their everyday life in terms of memory, comprehension, and manual dexterity."   (GE-4)

Another hard look at "mental deterioration" with age

A common notion, shared even by some physicians, has been that intellectual functioning reaches a peak in the late teens and thereafter begins a slow, but steady, decline.

But this is not the case at all, according to studies carried out by Dr. Lissy F. Jarvik, professor of psychiatry at the University of California, Los Angeles. Not only is there no falloff in knowledge or reasoning capacity into the thirties and forties, there is none into the seventies, and even eighties.

Among the studies was one begun with a group of people in their sixties who were checked and rechecked into their seventies and eighties; they experienced no intellectual decline although it did take them longer, as they grew older, to carry out intellectual functions.

Dr. Jarvik's studies also show that although older people often complain of poor memory, many learn as well as younger people, and their memory is also often equal. The studies indicate that much of what is thought to be memory loss may really be the result of inadequate learning caused by hearing difficulty, impaired vision, inattention, and similar factors.

Jarvik's work also indicates (and she emphasizes) that often what appears to be mental deterioration in an older person is a symptom of mental depression instead, and can be overcome by psychotherapy or antidepressant medication.   (GE-5)

An often-missed problem in older people

Giant cell arteritis, an artery inflammation that may occur after age fifty, may well explain some otherwise mysterious symptoms in older people, and, once diagnosed, the inflammation can be treated effectively.

Within the last half dozen years, studies have indicated that giant cell arteritis may affect one or more arteries in different areas of the body, producing a considerable range of symptoms—personality changes, headaches, rheumatism, fever, anemia, flulike discomfort, lassitude, appetite loss.

The cause of the inflammation is still unknown. One helpful clue to diagnosis is a high blood-sedimentation rate—the rate at which blood cells settle out of plasma.

The only effective treatment is corticosteroid therapy. A corticosteroid drug such as prednisone in a daily dose of 40 to 60 milligrams may bring improvement within twenty-four to forty-eight hours. The improvement, in fact, is often so dramatic that it is considered an important part of the diagnosis. Drug dosage may be reduced gradually over a period of several weeks and in some patients may be discontinued while others require low doses indefinitely.

Physicians active in arteritis research suggest that when older people begin to fail, giant cell arteritis should be one of the first rather than one of the last possible problems to be checked into.   (GE-6)

Ulcers after sixty

Far from being limited to vigorous younger people "on the make" in careers and society, although that's the popular conception, peptic ulcers can and do affect older people—and it is important that that fact be known if ulcer disease is to be recognized and treated in the elderly.

More than thirty recent studies of ulcer patients show that one of every six of those with chronic stomach ulcers and 5.1 percent of those with chronic duodenal ulcers experienced first symptoms after the age of sixty.

In addition to revealing that stomach ulcers are more of a geriatric problem than duodenal ulcers, the studies also indicate that stomach ulcer patients are more likely to delay seeking medical help than are those with duodenal ulcers.   (GE-7)

Treating cancer in older people

Is aggressive treatment, including major surgery, justified in elderly patients with limited life expectancy? Do the expected benefits of survival warrant the risk of operation?

A recent study of 226 patients with cancer of the colon or rectum, all of whom were at least eighty years of age, provides some answers.

Average life expectancy of eighty-year-old people in general is 6.4 years; at age eighty-five, it is 4.6 years. If people at advanced ages can be treated so that they can spend their remaining years in reasonable comfort, the contrast with the progressive deterioration and suffering of the patient with untreated cancer is stark.

All the 226 patients in the study had other coexisting diseases along with colorectal cancer. Yet their five-year survival rate after surgery for the cancer was 22.4 percent. The corresponding figure for all patients with colorectal cancer regardless of age was 24.2 percent. But considering other factors, regardless of cancer, influencing survival at various ages, the age-corrected survival rate of the elderly group with surgically treated cancer proved to be 53 percent. So that, the investigators report, it is possible to conclude that the relative prognosis of aged persons with surgically treated colorectal cancer is even more favorable than that of younger persons with the same disease.   (GE-8)

Surgery was used in 114 patients with lung cancer, all over the age of sixty-five, twenty-five of them in their seventies. As needed, they had surgery to remove either a whole affected lung or one or more lobes of a lung. Forty percent of the patients survived longer than four years. Most were content to be alive and to accept reduced lung function.

In contrast, survival statistics of patients over age sixty-five with lung cancer not undergoing surgery show only 2.7 percent surviving more than two years. Overall, patients over sixty-five with lung cancer appear to have a 77 percent chance of dying in the first six months and a 93 percent chance of dying within a year. Surgery in suitable cases, providing a 40 percent chance of survival for four years, appears justified, conclude the investigators.   (GE-9)

"No mandatory retirement from therapy?"

Within the last year, an editorial with that title appeared in the *Journal of the American Medical Association.*

Its thrust was this: That benefits of major surgical procedures are often withheld from older patients because of considerations of increased risk and decreased life expectancy. But "however important these considerations may be, they do not conceal an element of rationalization. One can detect an underlying assumption that the quality of life attainable in the elderly is poor at best, so that heroic attempts at improving handicaps and disabilities are hardly worthwhile."

Yet, the editorial pointed out, that such considerations are no longer tenable is attested to by recent reports on the increasing number of major surgical procedures carried out on older patients. "Clearly, surgical advances are catching up with advancing age."   (GE-10)

These are some of many reports recently on the results of surgery in elderly patients:

• Successful repair of hernia in 98 percent of two hundred patients, aged seventy and older, including two in their nineties.   (GE-11)

• A 98 percent chance of marked improvement or complete improvement after gallbladder and other biliary tract surgery in patients in the late sixties and older.   (GE-12)

• Increasing use at Massachusetts General Hospital of kidney transplants in older patients, including some in the late sixties, with a survival rate comparable to that for patients of all ages receiving kidney transplants.   (GE-13)

• Successful open heart surgery, including heart valve replacement in 84 percent of patients aged sixty-six or older.   (GE-14)

• Successful coronary bypass surgery in 90 percent of patients aged sixty-five or older, with long-term follow-up showing significant improvement in 93 percent of the survivors.   (GE-15)

CHAPTER 11

Headaches

A help for "cluster" headaches

Piercing, throbbing, pounding, splitting, or just dull headaches are virtually universal. It's estimated that seven of every ten adults use painkillers for headaches at least once a month, and for at least one of every twelve people headaches are a chronic problem.

One type of headache for which ordinary painkillers or analgesics and sometimes even expert medical treatment are of little value is a severe, one-sided one, involving eye, temple, neck, and face, with tearing of the eye and a thin, watery discharge from the nose.

It is called cluster because, characteristically, it may appear suddenly, be present every day for many days or weeks, disappear for a time, then return in another clustered batch.

At Stanford University, Stanford, California, Dr. Albert V. Giampaoli has reported promising results in treating cluster headaches with epinephrine (also known as adrenaline) administered in aerosol form. In a series of patients, three to six inhalations, fifteen to twenty minutes apart, usually broke the cyclic pattern, and when headaches did recur, the pain was much less intense.

One patient, for whom epinephrine alone was not adequate, had complete relief when another agent, ergotamine, frequently used for migraine, was added to the spray.   (H-1)

Relieving muscle-spasm headaches

When muscles anywhere go into spasm, or involuntary continuous contraction, pain can result. In turn, the pain leads to more contraction and the increased contraction to more pain, establishing a vicious cycle.

Headaches in many cases stem from anxiety, which leads to tension and spasmodic contraction of muscles at the base of the skull. A Canadian neurologist, Dr. H. M. Toupin of Edmonton, Alberta, has reported that in his experience, for 61 percent of patients with headaches severe enough to be sent for neurological study, the problem lies with emotionally induced muscle spasm.

Some patients, he has found, can be helped by restricting the intake of caffeine-containing beverages (coffee, tea, cola) to three or four cups a day and use of heat and massage. Prescribed tranquilizing or calmative agents such as diazepam sometimes are useful.

Despite such measures, however, some patients continue to have headaches and for them, the Canadian neurologist found, relief frequently can be obtained by injecting into the contracted muscles a mixture of a local anesthetic, lidocaine, and a cortisonelike agent such as methylprednisolone.   (H-2)

Migraine and diet

Hoping to avoid repeated attacks, many migraine sufferers resort to various diets, some of them bizarre (living, for example, primarily on such items as bananas and onions).

Despite a whole host of misconceptions about diet and migraine, reports Dr. Donald J. Dalessio of the University of Kentucky College of Medicine, some dietary measures may be helpful in many cases.

Certain foods can, in the migraine-prone, have an effect on blood vessels that may lead to attacks. They include red wines and champagne, aged or strong cheese (particularly cheddar), pickled herring, chicken livers, pods of broad beans, and canned figs. Their avoidance may be beneficial.

In some cases, cured meats, including frankfurters, bacon, ham, and salami, may have adverse effects and a trial of avoiding them may be worthwhile.

Monosodium glutamate in excessive amounts may trigger migraine and should be avoided.

It is also important, Dr. Dalessio reports, for migraine sufferers to avoid hypoglycemia, or low blood sugar. For this reason, they should eat three well-balanced meals a day, avoiding excessive amounts of sugar and starches at any one meal.   (H-3)

A tip on forecasting migraine—and when to take medication

The usual medications for migraine sometimes work, sometimes do not, as many sufferers know well. Important in determining success or failure is good or poor absorption of the medicine—and a nauseous stomach commonly absorbs medication poorly.

Advises one migraine expert, Dr. Walter C. Alvarez, emeritus professor at Mayo Clinic: Every migraine victim should be aware that if he or she waits to take antimigraine medication until nausea is already present, it may not be effective.

A valuable maneuver, which can help determine whether a migraine or an ordinary headache is coming on, he suggests, is to sit down and place the head between the knees. If the head then throbs, a migraine episode is on the way and medication for it should be taken immediately.   (H-4)

Migraine and estrogen

Is it possible that oral contraceptives and other preparations containing the hormone estrogen may play a role in migraine headaches in some women? So it seems from a study of three hundred patients with migraine carried out by Dr. Lee Kudrow of the California Medical Clinic for Headache in Encino.

According to Dr. Kudrow's report in the medical journal *Headache,* the estrogen-containing Pill and medications often increased headache frequency. In addition, they led to migrainelike headaches in some nonmigrainous women. And with elimination or reduction in dosage of the estrogen-containing preparations, a significant reduction in headache attack frequency occurred.   (H-5)

A heart drug to relieve migraine

Propranolol, a drug often used for heart patients, has turned out to have a dividend effect. Unexpectedly, some physicians using it for their heart patients noticed that a number of those who also happened to be migraine sufferers experienced relief for their headaches as well as their chest pains and other heart problems.

As the word got around and more and more physicians tried it for migraine patients without setting up scientifically controlled studies, the need for such studies became apparent. At the University of Miami, two neurologists, Drs. R. B. Weber and O. M. Reinmuth, set up such a study.

They chose nineteen patients with unyielding migraine, all failures on other treatment. Over a six-month period, they received propranolol in 20-milligram doses four times a day for three of the months and placebo (an inert, look-alike medication) the other three months with neither patients nor physicians knowing whether propranolol or placebo was being used at any given time, until the code was broken at the end of the study.

Propranolol proved to be helpful, indeed, for these patients with difficult migraine. The response of six of the nineteen was rated "excellent," with complete disappearance of the headaches after one week of propranolol treatment. Another nine had a "good" response—a 50 percent or greater reduction in the frequency or severity of attacks. Of the remaining four, two showed some improvement, two showed none at all.   (H-6)

Biofeedback for migraine and tension headaches

Biofeedback is, in effect, an extension of the normal way in which we learn. Learning is a process of getting "feedback" cues from such sources as our eyes, ears, hands, and feet. Swing at a golf club, for example, and you feel your arms move, see how the club connects with the ball, and where the ball goes—all cues to guide you to correcting your swing for possibly better ball placement next time.

Ordinarily, however, we get few feedback cues to what is going on inside the body. Sensitive electronic equipment can provide such awareness. With electrodes attached at various points on the body, the equipment can detect, amplify, and display small internal fluctuations in the form of sound beeps or light flashes, for example.

At the Menninger Foundation in Topeka, Kansas, one of the first institutions to study use of biofeedback for migraine, notable successes have been achieved by taping temperature sensors to a patient's finger and forehead. A meter shows the difference between head and hand temperature.

The patient, watching the meter, is asked to do such things as relax while repeating a calming phrase (for example, "I feel quiet") in order to relax blood vessels in the hands and thus increase hand temperature. When he or she succeeds, the meter needle moves. And with the relaxation and the warming of the hands comes a redistribution of blood that reduces pressure in blood vessels in the head, ending the migraine headache.

Once a patient develops the ability to move the needle, the same technique can be used, without the biofeedback equipment, to cut short a migraine attack.

Seventy-four percent of migraine sufferers have improved and have developed the ability to increase blood flow in the hands in almost 100 percent of the situations in which they detect the onset of a headache.

Biofeedback has also been found to work well for tension headaches—the most common kind, caused by contraction of forehead, scalp, and neck muscles—with improvement rates of up to 80 percent reported.

Hospitals now are beginning to use biofeedback in outpatient clinics for both types of headaches.

At one such hospital clinic, Long Island Jewish, for example, patients with tension headaches have sensor electrodes applied to the forehead to record muscle tension. If the level is high, the biofeedback machine emits a series of rapid beeps the patients hear through earphones. As tension is reduced, the beeps slow.

The device does two things, physicians at the clinic report. It gives a patient a precise measurement of his physical state as it pertains to his headaches. And it gives him the gratification of knowing he can alter that state. "In effect," they say, "the signal, beeping at the desired pace, tells the patient, 'You are in charge of yourself.' " (H-7)

Posttraumatic headaches

Headaches that develop after accidental injuries, especially injuries in the neck area, may stubbornly resist treatment with usual analgesics such as aspirin and acetaminophen (an aspirin substitute available under various trade names including Tylenol and Datril).

Often such headaches are accompanied by excessive sweating and dilation of the pupils of the eyes because the neck area injury has disturbed normal functioning of the nervous system.

At the University of California School of Medicine, Davis, Drs. N. Vijayan and P. M. Dreyfus have found that propranolol (see "A heart drug to relieve migraine," above) often produces prompt relief of such headaches after failure of all other medications, including ergotamine preparations. (H-8)

Cured meat headaches

Nitrites are chemical compounds that may be used as preservatives in cured meats. The compounds also are color fixers, helping to keep the meats looking red and fresh.

In some people sensitive to nitrites, however, they may be responsible for otherwise mysterious headaches.

One such case involved a fifty-eight-year-old man who for seven years experienced occasional moderately severe, nonthrobbing headaches. The attacks usually lasted several hours and were sometimes accompanied by facial flushing.

Finally, it became apparent that the attacks developed within half an hour after he ate such cured meat products as frankfurters, bacon, salami, and ham.

Since no other foods or beverages produced his headaches and he was not otherwise prone to headaches, tests to determine whether the nitrites in the cured meat products might be the culprits were carried out by Drs. William R. Henderson and Neil H. Raskin of the University of California at San Francisco department of neurology.

For the tests, he drank odorless, tasteless solutions that sometimes contained 10 milligrams of sodium nitrite and at other times contained the same amount of sodium bicarbonate. Headaches were provoked eight times out of the thirteen times he drank the sodium nitrite. (H-9)

Bedcover headaches

It would be difficult to think of a more unlikely cause of puzzling headaches than bedcovers—or, more accurately, sleeping with bedcovers pulled up over the head.

Yet that cause for headaches has been reported in the *Journal of the American Medical Association* by one investigative physician whose pet name for them is "turtle headaches."

The headaches may wake the victim during the night or may be present on awakening in the morning. They may be generalized, with pain all over the head, but usually they are most painful in front of the head.

They are accounted for, the physician suggests, by oxygen shortage resulting from the habit of pulling covers well up over the head. In his experience, once the cover-up habit is eliminated, so, immediately, are the headaches.   (H-10)

Depression headaches in childhood

Children are subject to many of the same types of headaches as adults.

Migraine is common although it often takes a little different form than in adults. Frequently in children, especially early in the development of the migraine pattern, there may be nausea and vomiting without the presence of any actual headache.

Tension or muscular contraction headaches are also common, especially during the school year.

Common, too, are inflammatory headaches associated with sinusitis, hay fever, and allergy.

And, just as do adults, children may suffer from headaches associated with mental depression. When the depression is recognized and treated, the headaches may clear.

In a study of twenty-five children with severe headaches, Dr. Walter Ling and other physicians of Washington University School of Medicine and Children's Hospital, Saint Louis, checked each child for a number of criteria: significant change of mood, social withdrawal, increasingly poor performance in school, disturbances of sleep, newly developed aggressive behavior, self-deprecation, lack of energy, weight loss, appetite loss, beliefs of persecution.

Any child found to have four or more of the criteria and not suffering from another psychiatric illness was considered to be depressed. Ten of the children qualified. The criteria most commonly present in the ten: mood change, social withdrawal, and self-deprecation.

When the children were treated with antidepressant medication such as amitriptyline or imipramine, their headaches as well as low mood benefited.   (H-11)

CHAPTER 12

Heart Disease

Each year, diseases of the heart and blood vessels take more than one million lives in the United States. They are the nation's leading cause of death.

Many studies have been and continue to be directed at establishing new insights into the factors involved in development of the diseases, and how they might be prevented, and into more effective methods of treatment.

Prevention

The likely victims

Why do some people, especially relatively young men, develop coronary heart disease and others not?

Studying more than thirteen hundred army men with the disease and comparing them with other men, National Academy of

Sciences-National Research Council investigators found that those who developed the disease with one or more of its manifestations— the chest pain of angina pectoris, heart attack, or death—had higher blood pressures, greater weight, heavier frame, and tended to be shorter in height.

More so than others, the men with heart disease tended to come from the Middle Atlantic states, to be of higher socioeconomic status, to have some graduate education and to be of officer rank, and also to be of Jewish origin and to have blood group A. There seemed to be a significantly lesser risk of coronary disease among men from rural areas and those whose earlier jobs had involved much physical activity.

About some of these factors, of course, nothing can be done. But like others, the investigation points to the importance of avoiding excessive weight, keeping blood pressure at normal levels, and being physically active.   (HT-1)

Another recent study has looked into the puzzling question of why some, but not all, people with coronary heart disease develop angina pectoris, with its chest pain, on exertion.

In Israel, at the University of Tel-Aviv Medical School, researchers selected from ten thousand men aged forty and over those who were free of angina and had not had heart attacks. Over a five-year period, during which the group was followed, some developed angina. And among factors significantly associated with the development were high blood pressure, high cholesterol level, diabetes, lack of physical activity, anxiety, peptic ulcer, and serious psychosocial problems.   (HT-2)

The effect of modifying diet

How effectively does a modification of diet reduce fat and cholesterol intake? And in particular for younger men who already have coronary heart disease?

In a study by investigators of the Atherosclerosis Research Group, Montclair, New Jersey, one hundred men, aged thirty to fifty, all with coronary heart disease and all with a history of heart attack, were placed on a low fat diet and matched with a group of comparable men not under dietary management.

Over the ten-year period of the study, the diet-managed men experienced marked reductions in blood-fat levels compared with the others and, at the end of the ten years, had a 17 percent greater survival rate.   (HT-3)

Can artery disease be reversed?

Some hope that already-present artery clogging can be reversed comes from animal studies at the University of Chicago by Drs. Draga Vesselinovitch and Robert W. Wissler.

After feeding monkeys high cholesterol diets for eighteen months, the two researchers sacrificed some of the animals and, upon autopsy, found extensive coronary and other artery disease.

They then divided the remaining monkeys into two groups, some remaining on a high cholesterol-fat diet while others were placed on a low fat diet. Later, upon sacrifice, the animals on the low fat diet had markedly fewer fatty deposits on their artery linings than did the others, suggesting to the investigators that "to some degree, even advanced stages of the disease can be reversed if sufficiently low blood cholesterol levels are sustained for a long period of time." (HT-4)

A new view: the role of overnutrition

Is it the type of diet or the amount in the diet that counts most in holding cholesterol and blood-fat levels down? An answer now comes from a study of 4,057 adults in Tecumseh, Michigan, by Drs. Allen B. Nichols and Leon D. Ostrander of the University of Michigan School of Medicine.

For each of the participating adults, tallies were made of consumption of 110 different food items; of average consumption of foods high in fat, starch, sugar, and alcohol; and of total daily caloric intake.

For both men and women in the study, it turned out that cholesterol and blood-fat levels did not correlate particularly well with the kind of diet but it did with body fat. The study, the investigators report, suggests that overnutrition—too much caloric intake leading to weight gain and body-fat accumulation—is more important in raising blood levels than the proportions of fat, starch, sugar, or alcohol in the diet.   (HT-5)

Exercise, blood fats, and heart disease

Can exercise—vigorous exercise—make a major difference in

blood-fat levels and health of the heart? Two recent studies shed some light on this.

In Palo Alto, California, where Stanford University has a Heart Disease Prevention Program, Drs. Peter D. Wood and William Haskell studied forty-one men, ranging in age from thirty-five to fifty-nine, who averaged fifteen miles of running per week. Many had only begun to run in the last few years.

Blood-fat levels in these men were more like those of young women least vulnerable to heart disease than those of sedentary middle-aged men. Blood cholesterol levels were significantly lower and blood-fat (triglyceride) levels were only half those of men of comparable age leading sedentary lives.

No runner smoked cigarettes; almost all were close to ideal weight. Still, the investigators believe, the study indicates that exercising, rather than the other factors, was primarily responsible for the healthy blood levels. Caution the investigators emphatically: No vigorous program of exercise should *ever* be undertaken without adequate progressive conditioning and medical advice.   (HT-6)

In Great Britain, another study covered 16,882 business executives, aged forty to sixty-four, who reported their exercise habits in response to a questionnaire. Subsequently 232 of the men suffered a first attack of coronary heart disease. Analysis of the questionnaires showed that light exercise provided no special advantage, but among those men who had reported vigorous exercise habits, the risk of developing heart disease was only one-third that for other men. (HT-7)

Water and the heart

A role for soft water in heart attacks and strokes has been suggested by many studies. In Monroe County, Florida, for example, after the local water supply was converted from soft rain to hard well water, heart attack and stroke death rates were halved over a four-year period.

Although the mechanism by which soft water increases risk is not established, two possibilities have been proposed: that soft water may in some way affect the heart muscle directly or that it tends to favor high blood pressure, which is usually more prevalent in soft water areas.

Some investigators now suggest that although hard drinking water in itself may not by any means guarantee reduced risk of heart attack or stroke, those living in hard water areas who soften their water may do well to leave at least one tap producing hard water for drinking purposes.   (HT-8)

High blood pressure

High blood pressure, or hypertension, affects upwards of twenty-three million Americans, and is now recognized to be a major factor not only in heart disease but also in strokes and kidney failure.

What makes it so major a factor, even when it produces no obvious symptoms, is the effect of elevated pressure over a prolonged period of time on arteries in different parts of the body.

Under the constant bombardment of abnormal pressure, the arteries become thickened and arteriosclerotic. As these changes occur, the heart muscle itself is affected by the burden of having to pump harder against the higher pressure. It first becomes enlarged to do the pumping but in time it loses pumping efficiency. With the reduced efficiency, blood circulation becomes impaired, leading to congestive failure—with fluid accumulation and congestion occurring in body organs. The legs become swollen; so do the lungs; heart pain, or angina, may appear and so may a heart attack.

Increased pressure over many years may also damage the kidneys, leading to kidney failure. Increased pressure in brain blood vessels over an extended period may lead to stroke.

The first conclusive evidence of the value of treating hypertension in reducing heart disease, strokes, and other deadly problems came from studies late in the sixties and early in the seventies by a Veterans Administration Cooperative Study Group. The studies indicated that even in patients with relatively moderate hypertension, the risk of developing serious complications over a five-year period was reduced from 55 percent to 18 percent by treatment. With treatment, the incidence of stroke was reduced fourfold, and heart failure and kidney deterioration did not occur over the five years.

In almost every case today, hypertension can be treated effectively by drugs and, in some cases, by diet emphasizing weight reduction and reduced salt intake.

The effectiveness of treatment has begun to lead to a change in attitude among insurance companies, which, until recently, either refused insurance for hypertensives or issued it only at stiff extra premium cost.

One late study by an insurance company, Aetna Life and Casualty, has found that treated hypertensives have a 50 to 100 percent lower death rate in every disease category than the untreated. As a result, insurance for hypertensives is increasingly available.   (HT-9, 10)

Type A behavior

In recent years, a pattern of behavior that is significantly related to coronary heart disease has been reported by Drs. Meyer Friedman and Ray H. Rosenman of San Francisco, and others.

Called Type A behavior, it is characterized by excessive drive, ambition, and competitiveness, and by a strong sense of time urgency. In contrast to Type A individuals, Type B people are not, by any means, necessarily passive, unproductive, or unsuccessful, but they are not excessively driven, not excessively competitive, and are free, relatively, of a sense of time urgency.

Based on an eight-and-a-half-year study of 3,500 men, Friedman and Rosenman have reported that Type A individuals are more than twice as prone to coronary heart disease, five times more prone to a second heart attack, and have fatal heart attacks twice as frequently.

In the latest study, carried out by investigators of the University of Western Ontario in Canada with managers from twelve different companies, of whom over 61 percent were found to be Type A, additional facts were determined.

Type A individuals were found to have significantly higher blood pressure, and higher cholesterol and blood-fat levels. A greater percentage were cigarette smokers. They were also less interested in and participated less in exercise and physical activity.

For an average man at age forty-five, the probability of developing coronary heart disease in the next six years has been shown to be 4.4 percent. The Canadian investigators report that Type A individuals, because of their higher number of such risk factors as elevated pressure, smoking, and high cholesterol and blood-fat levels, have a 6.3 percent probability, or about a 50 percent greater risk, of coronary heart disease.   (HT-11)

Treatment

Newer insights into heart attacks: real death causes and delays

In the next hour, as things now stand, some 125 Americans will experience heart attacks and many will die needlessly—because of failure to recognize that the attacks are occurring or hesitation in seeking immediate treatment.

A heart attack can be massive, with so much of the heart muscle destroyed that there is no chance for life. But far more often it is not that massive and may even be quite mild, yet death may occur within the first few hours because of electrical failure.

In a heart attack, with obstruction in a coronary artery blocking blood flow to a portion of the heart muscle, very often a small portion, electrical patterns in the heart, which determine heart rhythm, may be disturbed temporarily, leading to abnormal rhythms.

Today, in a hospital, even the most serious, potentially fatal, rhythm abnormalities often can be corrected and, in fact, with monitoring equipment, early warnings of the abnormalities can be picked up and medications can be used to prevent them from occurring.

Unfortunately, more than half of the six hundred thousand Americans who succumb to heart attacks each year do so before ever getting to a hospital where their chances for survival would be significantly improved.

Some recent studies have shown an average elapsed time of three and a half hours between start of symptoms of heart attack and hospitalization, with delay in some cases stretching to as long as five days.

In some cases, the delay stems from reluctance to seek help even though the attack is recognized for what it is, perhaps because of failure to understand the value of immediate treatment.

Often, however, the problem lies with failure to recognize the heart attack and attributing the experience to gas pains, diabetes, gallbladder disease, and even, some studies indicate, the common cold.

(HT-12)

Recognizing the symptoms—and acting

The most common symptom of a heart attack is chest pain. In some cases, there is a feeling of unusual discomfort or pressure in the center of the chest, behind the breastbone; in others, the feeling is one of the chest being crushed in a vise. Sometimes, the pain may radiate, spreading into the throat, shoulders, arms, or back.

In some cases, the chest pain may be accompanied by a feeling of great anxiety and a sense of nearness of death. The face may turn ashen gray.

Nausea, vomiting, sweating, and shortness of breath may also be present in some cases.

A heart attack may occur without previous warning of anything wrong with the heart. It may also occur in people who are well aware they have a heart problem because of episodes of angina pectoris or chest pain on exertion.

Angina patients have been known to become confused and to think that a heart attack is another angina episode. But where the chest pain of angina stops quickly after activity ceases or after nitroglycerin is taken, the chest pain of a heart attack does not.

There is only one safe way to proceed when chest pain occurs or when, in an angina patient, it occurs and does not disappear with rest or nitroglycerin: get to a physician. This commonly means getting to a hospital emergency room.

Added help for the heart attack

A wide variety of measures, ranging from pain relieving agents, oxygen, and anticlotting drugs to chemicals to strengthen the heart and improve its function and compounds to prevent or overcome serious rhythm abnormalities can be used as needed for heart attack patients.

Now, in studies in more than twenty medical centers, a new procedure has been found to halve the mortality associated with moderately severe heart attacks.

It involves encasing the patient's legs in special "bootlike" equipment and applying pressure to the large blood vessel bed in the legs. The pressure is synchronized so that it is exerted during diastole, the period between heart beats. When exerted at that point, it increases the blood flow through the coronary arteries that feed the heart muscle.

The technique was developed at Tufts-New England Medical Center, Boston, by Dr. John S. Banas. In the multiple-medical center study, the technique was used in 108 of 224 patients and results were compared with those for the remaining 116 patients who received conventional treatment.

In those patients receiving "external pressure circulatory assist (EPCA)," as the technique is known, in-hospital mortality was 7 percent contrasted with 15 percent in the others. Only 1 percent of

EPCA treated patients had ventricular fibrillation, a potentially deadly rhythm abnormality, versus 7 percent of the others.   (HT-13)

After an attack: early activity

Where once it was the custom to keep patients in bed for extended periods after a heart attack, now the tendency is to abbreviate the bed rest period and encourage early activity for patients who have no complications.

In one recent study by Dr. A. Bloch and a medical team at Hôpital Cantonal, Geneva, Switzerland, 154 patients free of complications on the first or second day after their attack were randomly assigned to two groups for comparison. One underwent the traditional period of strict bed rest for three or more weeks. The other group were placed on a program of progressive activity.

For the active patients, the mean duration of hospital stay was 21.3 days; for the others, 32.8. There were no significant differences between the two groups in heart attack recurrence rates, heart failure, or chest pain attacks, but, on follow-up study over a period of six to twenty months, the strict bed-rest group had greater disability than did the active group.   (HT-14)

When coronary bypass surgery may be valuable

A coronary circulation system supplies the heart muscle with blood and nutrients. The system consists of three main coronary arteries and their branches.

With coronary artery disease that leads to anginal chest pain and heart attack, a part or several parts of the system become choked up with fatty deposits so that the inner bore is narrowed, reducing blood flow to the heart muscle, or in some cases a section of the system becomes completely obstructed.

In the last ten years a surgical technique of bypassing blocks in the coronary circulation has come into increasing use. Usually a length of saphenous vein is used. The vein is a large vessel running the length of each leg, but it can be spared because other veins can take over its work; this is the vein commonly removed in varicose vein surgery.

The vein section is attached to the body's main trunkline artery, the aorta, and then connected to a coronary artery at a point beyond where it is obstructed. More than one such bypass—even as many as six and eight—may be performed for an individual patient.

The operation is formidable. At first the operative death rate ran about 14 percent. This has now been greatly reduced and, depending upon an individual patient's problems, the risk may be as little as 1 or 2 percent.

When is coronary bypass surgery really needed? When is it likely to be more effective than medical management in improving the outlook for survival? There has been contention between cardiologists and heart surgeons, which is not likely to be entirely resolved until the results of many long-term studies are in.

But experiences accumulated to date suggest that certain patients may do best with surgery. It appears that patients who benefit most—those for whom surgery can make a lifesaving difference—are those with blocking of at least two of the main coronary arteries or of the left main coronary artery alone. This may amount to about half of all patients with angina.

Among the studies indicating this is one by Dr. Nicholas T. Kouchoukos of the University of Alabama. In that study, bypass surgery was performed on eighty-five patients with at least 50 percent closing-off of their left main coronary artery. Eighty-seven percent are alive after two years, contrasted with 62 percent survival among comparable patients treated medically. None of the medicated patients was ever completely free of angina; about 60 percent of the bypass group were pain-free after the operation. Kouchoukos's experience also indicates that two-year results with bypasses for two or more main arteries are equally good.

Another study supporting the Alabama experience has been made at the Veterans Administration hospital in Oteen, North Carolina, by Dr. Timothy Takaro. In more than a hundred patients with at least 50 percent blockage of the left main coronary artery who received either surgery or medical treatment, the two-year mortality among those medically treated was 38 percent, but after bypass surgery it was 17 percent.   (HT-15)

Surgery for congenital heart defects

Among children with congenital heart defects operated on recently at Boston Children's Hospital Medical Center was an infant boy only thirty-six hours old with a potentially deadly defect.

After he was anesthetized, his body was covered with a plastic blanket and the blanket in turn was covered with cracked ice. When his body temperature had fallen to 77 degrees, the infant's chest was opened and he was hooked up to a heart-lung machine that pumped gradually cooled blood through his body until his temperature was down to 68. At that point, the pump could be turned off and the child lay in a state of suspended animation, his heart motionless, and all circulation stopped.

Surgeons then went to work, using magnifying spectacles, to rearrange the abnormally placed blood vessels from lungs to heart. When that was completed in an hour, the pump was turned on again and rewarmed blood was circulated through the baby's body. The newly repaired heart soon began beating again.

Such total body chilling, also called deep hypothermic circulatory arrest, to permit open-heart surgery, extends further the ability of surgeons to help children born with heart defects.

Each year in the United States, thirty thousand to forty thousand babies are born with such defects, not all of them serious, some of them even self-correcting over a period of time, many manageable with medical measures. But some defects are very serious, may interfere with growth and development, cause suffering and invalidism, shorten life expectancy, or even threaten life almost immediately.

With recent advances in surgical techniques, anesthesia, and support for children before, during, and after surgery, success rates for some of these operations are as high as 99 percent.

In many cases of congenital defects that need surgical correction, there need be no immediate urgency. The operations often can be delayed safely to age five or even to age ten or twelve. They are often technically easier to perform then.

In cases where a child urgently needed surgery much earlier, palliative procedures often were used—relatively simple and safe techniques for tiding the child over until later the definitive surgery could be performed.

But sometimes palliative procedures have had drawbacks, exposing a child to the risk of two operations, for example, and sometimes allowing the child's growth to be impaired while awaiting the definitive procedure.

Very recently, with increasing success, surgeons have been performing definitive rather than palliative surgery at earlier and earlier ages. And recently, the use of deep hypothermia has made it possible in some very seriously affected children for successful repairs to be carried out very early in life, even just hours after birth.   (HT-16)

CHAPTER 13

Neurologic Disorders

New help for the burning pain of causalgia

Causalgia, the result of irritation to or injury of a nerve, produces a burning pain, in some cases so persistent and severe that sympathectomy, a nerve-cutting operation, has been needed.

Now comes a first report of use of a drug, propranolol, originally employed for heart conditions, with striking benefits for patients scheduled for sympathectomy. The report has been made by Dr. George Simson of Albuquerque, New Mexico.

In one case, a woman with unyielding causalgia of her foot, who had experienced minimal relief from increasing quantities of narcotics and had been on the verge of addiction after three months, had great relief within forty-eight hours after beginning to take propranolol; in the following week she could stop narcotics without further difficulty.

In another case, a man who had been bedfast because of causalgia after a trivial injury was completely relieved of pain within twelve hours and able to bear weight and become ambulatory within twenty-four hours.   (N-1)

For cerebral palsy babies: a new approach

A cooperative study under way at the Greater New Orleans Cerebral Palsy Center, the Meeting Street School Children's Rehabilitation Center in Providence, Rhode Island, and other centers concerned with cerebral palsy children is showing encouraging results of an approach to treatment that emphasizes active early intervention by parents and doctors.

Where once CP children were simply allowed to lie without moving their muscles, leading to paralysis, weakness, and tightness of muscles, now, with early activation of sensorimotor functions, children are developing less spasticity and distortion of movement, and need fewer complex surgical procedures later.

Procedures used include twirling and rolling babies to improve "body awareness." Mothers are encouraged as early as possible to touch, cuddle, and whisper to CP babies, to help them chew, and to use mobiles, hand puppets, and other devices to reinforce the children's vision and eye-hand coordination.

At the pioneering centers, varied specialists provide stimulation and enrichment programs.

It appears that some physicians, reluctant to inform parents early that their baby may be disabled and hoping that somehow the infant will outgrow early indications of abnormal development, may make a big mistake if they delay referring a baby to a suitable center.

Encouragingly, some doctors are beginning to make such referrals right from the intensive care hospital nursery without any delays and the study may help convince all physicians of the wisdom of doing the same.   (N-2)

A new treatment for childhood movement disorders (dystonia)

A first report indicates that Tegretol, a drug sometimes employed for the facial nerve disorder trigeminal neuralgia may be helpful for at least some children with dystonic movement disorders.

Tried in a group of eight children, four with hereditary torsion and four with acquired dystonia, the drug, in doses of 300 to 1,200 milligrams daily, has produced sustained improvement of some manifestations of the illness in every case for periods thus far of up to one year, report Dr. Martin Geller and other physicians at Mount Sinai School of Medicine, New York City.

Among the children responding well to the treatment: a thirteen-year-old boy who had been subject to as many as forty attacks a day of grimacing of the right side of the face and twisting of the trunk; a sixteen-year-old girl who had been suffering from uncontrollable spasms of trunk and legs and posturing of the hands; a five-and-one-half-year-old boy who had been subject to frequent falls because of violent spasms of his right leg and foot.   (N-3)

Treating nervous system diseases (neuropathies) by reducing high blood-fat levels

The woman was one of a small group of patients with bizarre symptoms seen at the Baylor College of Medicine department of neurology in Houston. She was fifty-seven, a successful real estate agent until two years before, when she had begun to suffer from irritability, depression, anxiety, unnecessary crying, and failing memory. She subsequently began to have other problems—dizzy spells, lack of coordination, tingling and numbness in both feet and occasionally in her fingers and hands.

She was checked for diabetes, cirrhosis, hypothyroidism, pancreatitis, and other disorders that might account for her troubles. She had none of these. But her blood-fat levels—cholesterol at 600 and triglycerides at 1,600—were greatly elevated.

It took a combination of diet and a medication, clofibrate, to bring her triglyceride level down to 183 and cholesterol to 217 over a period of three months. At that point, all her symptoms disappeared.

In five other patients seen at Baylor, similar symptoms—a kind of hyperlipidemic (high blood-fat level) dementia—yielded to diet alone to bring down the excessive levels.

How the excessive levels can produce the neuropathies or nervous system problems is unknown. "But the fact that patients improve when their hyperlipidemia is treated," say the Baylor neurologists, "makes it desirable to look for this defect in all patients with dementia and treat it as soon as it's found."   (N-4)

Epilepsy: newer treatments

Tranxene. Recently introduced into the United States after use in Europe, Tranxene gives promise of helping some patients with seizures that resist treatment with standard antiepileptic agents.

In one of its first United States trials—at the Epilepsy Center of the University of Wisconsin Center for Health Sciences, Madison—fifty-nine such patients received the drug. In twenty, seizures were greatly reduced in number or completely eliminated. Twelve of the twenty also experienced marked improvement in alertness, attention span, and school performance. Four others showed partial improvement in seizure control. Thirty-five were not helped. Tranxene proved to be helpful only when used in conjunction with other drugs; in no case did it control seizures when used alone.   (N-5)

Zarontin for petit mal. Occurring predominantly in children, petit mal or "absence" seizures commonly last only a few seconds during which a child blanks out briefly, stops any activity, then resumes it after the episode is over.

A particularly valuable drug for such seizures is Zarontin which, in studies by investigators at the National Institutes of Health, Bethesda, Maryland, proved capable of providing 50 percent to 100 percent control in 95 percent of children, with the seizures eliminated completely in 19 percent, and 90 percent or better control achieved in 49 percent. The drug did not produce drowsiness or impair performance on psychological testing.   (N-6)

Tegretol for grand mal and psychomotor epilepsy. In addition to its use for trigeminal neuralgia and more recently for children with dystonic movement disorders (see above), Tegretol has been used in other countries for more than a decade to treat epilepsy.

Recently, after studies here by investigators supported by the National Institutes of Health, the drug has been approved for use in epilepsy by the United States Food and Drug Administration.

Based on the United States studies, the drug is being called the first major advance in long-term treatment of grand mal and psychomotor epilepsy in two decades. It has been found to help some patients whose seizures have not been controlled at all or only partially controlled by such drugs as diphenylhydantoin, phenobarbital, or primidone.   (N-7)

Imipramine. A drug developed for combatting mental depression, imipramine may help some patients with petit mal and minor motor seizures who do not benefit from or stop benefiting from standard anticonvulsant agents.

Of twenty such patients studied by investigators at the University of Pittsburgh School of Medicine, fifteen responded well to imipramine.   (N-8)

Dextroamphetamine. This central nervous system stimulant, often used for treating narcolepsy (uncontrollable recurrent attacks of desire for sleep), can be of great benefit for some patients with epilepsy, according to studies at a major seizure center, the Samuel Livingstone Epilepsy Diagnostic and Treatment Center, Baltimore.

Investigators there report that the drug can help overcome the drowsiness induced by many anticonvulsant drugs, permitting patients to function well, and frequently makes possible use of very large doses of anticonvulsants needed for controlling seizures but otherwise impossible to use because of extreme drowsiness.

They also report that amphetamine alone is sometimes effective in controlling petit mal and myoclonic epilepsy, and, when taken at bedtime in a 5-milligram sustained release capsule for children and a 15-milligram sustained release capsule for adults, it is the most effective drug for controlling sleep seizures that often resist standard anticonvulsants.   (N-9)

Vitamin D. Can vitamin D be of any value for controlling seizures? A suggestion that it may be comes from a small-scale study at Glostrup Hospital in Denmark. Twenty-three patients, all on anticonvulsant medication for periods of three to seventeen years, took part. Over an eighty-four-day period, while usual medication was continued, some patients also received vitamin D and, for comparison, others received a look-alike but inert preparation.

The vitamin did have an additive effect, helping to reduce the number of seizures, although how it does so is unknown.   (N-10)

A dividend of effective treatment. When anticonvulsant medications work well to stop seizures, they may also produce improvement in mental and motor performance.

At the University of Ottawa, Canada, in a study by Dr. Ronald Trites, a group of epileptic children with a mean age of sixteen years received before and during treatment a battery of forty-seven tests to measure verbal and performance IQ, concept formation, speech perception, and motor and sensory functions including movement coordination and fine manipulative skills.

In two-thirds of the children whose seizures were controlled, scores on the test battery improved significantly.   (N-11)

The good long-term outlook for children with epilepsy. Two studies suggest that many children with various types of epilepsy who respond well to anticonvulsant drugs may after a period of time of freedom from seizures continue to do well without further medication.

At Washington University-Saint Louis Children's Hospital, Dr. Jean Holowach-Thurston and a medical team did a long-term follow-up study of 148 children whose medication had been tapered off to nothing after four seizure-free years. Seventy-six percent continued to be free of seizures without need for medication. Among those who experienced recurrences, the most critical time was the first year after stopping medication. Children with grand mal had a relapse rate of only 8 percent; those with febrile, or fever, seizures, 12 percent; petit mal, 12 percent; psychomotor, 25 percent. Among those with Jacksonian seizures of localized origin, however, the relapse rate was 53 percent, and children with more than one type of epilepsy had a 40 percent relapse rate.   (N-12)

At the University of Pittsburgh School of Medicine, Drs. G. H. Fromm and I. Chamovitz followed twenty-eight patients who first developed grand mal seizures between the ages of four and eight years. Twelve years later, only four were still experiencing seizures. Sixteen had been able to discontinue medication when they were seven to fourteen years of age without further difficulty; eight others had no more seizures at all after the first one for which they were treated.

It appears that the brain may be much more prone to seizures in childhood, and in some cases convulsions may occur only at this time.   (N-13)

The movement disorder: hemiballismus

Hemiballismus is a violent motor restlessness of half of the body, with continuous, flailing, involuntary movements most marked in the arm on the affected side but also occurring to a lesser degree in the leg on the same side.

Medical treatment has not helped and brain surgery has been

required. A first case of response to medication—haloperidol, one of a new series of tranquilizers—has been reported by Dr. Gordon J. Gilbert of the University of South Florida School of Medicine, Tampa.

Although extended study with many patients will be needed before the efficacy of the drug can be evaluated, the first patient began to show improvement within forty-eight hours after treatment with haloperidol was tried, and the improvement has been maintained with continued use of a reduced amount of the drug.   (N-14)

For myoclonus: a hopeful development

Myoclonus is a neurologic disorder leading to uncontrollable tremors of muscles at unpredictable times. The disorder may develop after accidental or other injury; it sometimes is familial; it may also accompany epilepsy in some cases.

A drug known as L-5-hydroxytryptophan (L-5-HTP) has been tried in the past but it so often produces severe nausea, diarrhea, and vomiting that it could not be used in large enough doses to be effective.

Recently, however, a combination of L-5-HTP in large doses and another drug, caridopa, in small amounts, has proved valuable in a small series of patients treated by Dr. Melvin H. VanWoert of Mount Sinai School of Medicine, New York City.

Among the patients, for example, a forty-seven-year-old man unable to shave, eat, or dress experienced complete disappearance of tremors four weeks after beginning the combination drug treatment. Another, a twenty-two-year-old woman with myoclonus associated with epilepsy, previously unable to speak, feed herself, or stand, or in fact do little more than breathe, has responded to the extent thus far of being able to eat well, stand on her own, and speak a few words. (N-15)

Myasthenia gravis

A nerve disorder that weakens muscles, myasthenia gravis may occur in either sex at any age but is most common in young adult women.

Its victims commonly experience abnormal fatigability and weakness, in particular, of muscles of the neck, throat, lips, tongue, face, and eyes. Many complain of double vision and difficulty in swallowing, chewing, and talking.

Drug treatments. Although drugs rarely produce complete elimination of symptoms, such drugs as neostigmine and pyridostigmine are often helpful. Now several recent studies suggest that in some patients for whom the usual drug treatment is inadequate, prednisone, a cortisonelike compound, may be valuable.

When prednisone was tried in the past, it often increased weakness. But at Johns Hopkins Hospital, Baltimore, Drs. Marjorie E. Seybold and Daniel B. Brachman have used prednisone in a group of twelve patients, starting with low doses (25 milligrams on alternate days) which were gradually increased to 100 milligrams every other day.

Ten of the twelve patients improved, with three of them virtually free of all symptoms. As yet, the Hopkins physicians report, there is no way to forecast which myasthenia patients will benefit and which will not.   (N-16)

Prednisone has been recently used too, with success, in a small group of patients for whom the most pronounced symptom of myasthenia was eye muscle weakness unresponsive to other medication. Of eight receiving prednisone every other day, seven have shown marked improvement, report Drs. K. C. Fischer and R. J. Schwartzman of Miami.   (N-17)

Surgery. Although the cause of myasthenia gravis is unknown, the thymus, a gland in the neck area, seems to have something to do with it. In some cases, a thymoma, or tumor of the gland may be present; in others, no tumor is present.

When a tumor is present or in some cases when medical control is poor, thymectomy—removal of the thymus gland—may be valuable.

At the University of California at Los Angeles Medical Center, Dr. D. G. Mulder and other investigators have followed one hundred patients selected for thymectomy because of poor medical control of the disease or the presence of tumor. Significant improvement occurred in fifty-two of fifty-eight women and ten of fifteen men who did not have thymoma and in twelve of sixteen women and five of eleven men who did have thymic tumor.   (N-18)

Other insights into the effects of surgery have come from recent studies. At Mount Sinai Hospital, New York City, a team headed by

Dr. A. E. Papatestas studied 185 patients undergoing thymectomy. They found that improvement does not usually take place in immediate dramatic fashion. There was an interval of two or more years before half of the 185 patients were completely freed of symptoms. After five years, 90 percent of the patients had improved or were completely free of symptoms.   (N-19)

Falling episodes

Mysterious falling episodes—falling forward or backward, while walking or standing—could in some cases be the result of parkinsonism, or shaking palsy, even when none of the typical signs of parkinsonism, such as stooped, shuffling gait and tremor at rest, are present.

Over a three-year period, eleven such patients were seen by Dr. H. L. Klawans of Michael Reese Medical Center and Dr. J. L. Topel of Rush-Presbyterian-Saint Luke's Medical Center, Chicago.

For the falling episodes, nine responded to treatment with amantadine, a drug frequently used for parkinsonism. In those failing to respond initially to amantadine or to continue to respond to it, another anti-parkinsonism agent, levadopa, proved effective.   (N-20)

Additional help for parkinsonism

Although helpful for many patients with parkinsonism, levadopa fails to benefit at least one-fourth. Many of the latter may be helped when an amphetamine drug—either dextroamphetamine sulfate or methylphenidate hydrochloride—is combined with levadopa treatment.

At Maimonides Medical Center, Brooklyn, New York, Drs. Edith Miller and H. A. Neiburg treated thirty such patients with amphetamine, achieving a significant improvement in gait. An additional twenty-one patients received methylphenidate for lethargy and somnolence induced by levadopa, and all were relieved of these side effects.

Amphetamines, it should be noted, must be used with caution in patients with some heart or psychiatric problems.   (N-21)

Relief for post-shingles neuralgia

Caused by the same herpes virus responsible for chickenpox, shingles is an acute infection of the nervous system, with neuralgic pain and skin outbreak during the acute period. In some cases, it may leave severe residual neuralgic pain after acute infection subsides, and the post-shingles neuralgia may persist for months or years.

A hopeful note is sounded by Dr. Arthur Taub of Yale University School of Medicine, New Haven, Connecticut. In a study with patients with post-shingles neuralgia, almost complete relief of pain followed within one to two weeks after the start of treatment with a combination of drugs—amitriptyline, a compound often used for mental depression, and a tranquilizing agent, such as perphenazine, fluphenazine, or thioridazine, often used for anxiety. Neither drug was effective when used alone.   (N-22)

Stroke

A major cause of stroke is obstruction of the carotid arteries (on either side of the neck), which are major avenues of blood circulation to the brain. The obstruction, produced by fatty deposits on the artery wall, reduces the vital blood flow and may lead to brain cell death.

Before a paralyzing or deadly stroke, many people have "little strokes"—momentary episodes of stumbling, numbness or paralysis of a hand, vision blurring, or speech or memory loss—indicative of reduced blood flow to the brain. As many as 50 percent of those who have such episodes go on to have a major stroke.

Until relatively recently, it was believed that most obstructions leading to stroke occurred in arteries buried within the brain and unreachable by surgery, with only a small minority occurring in the carotid circulation where they are available to surgery. Recent studies, however, indicate that as many as 74 percent of patients have at least one lesion at a surgically accessible site.

Carotid endarterectomy—a procedure in which a carotid artery is opened and the obstruction surgically scraped out—is highly effective in the treatment of patients with evidence of obstruction, relieving symptoms in most cases and markedly reducing the incidence of subsequent massive strokes, reports Dr. Jesse E. Thompson of Baylor University Medical Center, Dallas, on the basis of experience with more than 1,100 such procedures.   (N-23)

Simple tests. When there is suspicion that a carotid artery obstruction may be present, arteriography—which involves X-ray studies after injection into the artery of a contrast material or dye—is effective in spotting the obstruction. Arteriography entails some risk because of possible reaction to the contrast material, but is well justified when suspicion is serious.

Ideally, a safe, simple, noninvasive technique is needed for screening patients who *may* have obstruction. Two such tests have been reported recently.

One, called carotid compression tonography, measures pressure inside the eyeball (with an instrument similar to what is employed routinely for glaucoma detection) at the same time the examiner applies slight pressure on one side of the neck, just above the collarbone, for about four seconds. In studies with more than 350 patients, Dr. Richard Wangelin and other physicians at the Cleveland Clinic Foundation have found the test capable of successfully picking out 94 percent of those with serious obstruction of the carotid arteries. (N-24)

Another test involves simply placing a special stethoscopelike instrument on the forehead just above the eye. The electronic device permits an examiner to hear and record sound waves of blood flowing through a surface artery, and the sound wave pattern reveals the condition of the carotid arteries. At the University of California at Los Angeles School of Medicine, Drs. H. I. Machlader and W. F. Barker have used the test to detect obstruction in patients with premonitory stroke symptoms.

High blood pressure and stroke. High blood pressure is a leading cause of stroke and the higher the pressure, the greater the stroke risk. Even mild elevation of pressure, if undetected and untreated, can produce stroke, as shown in a Veterans Administration study of 523 men with diastolic blood pressure of 90 (the top normal) or higher. Among those not treated for mild elevations, twenty-five developed strokes as compared to six among those receiving treatment for the pressure elevation. With hypertension affecting upward of twenty-three million Americans, only about half of whom are aware they have elevated pressure, and only half of those who are aware being treated at all or being treated adequately, the study underscores the need for more awareness of the importance of hypertension detection and treatment.   (N-25)

High blood pressure after a stroke. Once a stroke occurs, does controlling elevated pressure do any good? In a study of 162 hypertensive patients who had recovered from stroke, investigators of the Medical Research Council Blood Pressure Unit, Western Infirmary, Glasgow, Scotland, found that the better the control of elevated pressure, the less likelihood of a stroke recurrence. Moreover, hypertension is often a factor in heart failure, and the frequency of failure was significantly higher in patients with poor control of hypertension.   (N-26)

Other aids for preventing stroke. A stroke-prevention program at Pennsylvania Hospital, Philadelphia, has demonstrated that major strokes can be largely avoided after little strokes have occurred.

In patients entering the program after a first little stroke, any and all high-risk factors—high blood pressure, excessive blood-fat levels, diabetes, obesity, stress, cigarette smoking, carotid artery obstruction—were identified and treated with medication, diet, avoidance of cigarettes where smoking was a factor, and, in about one-sixth of the patients, surgery to clear artery obstruction.

In a five-year follow-up period, only 6.6 percent of the patients—instead of an expectable 50 percent—experienced major strokes, only one-third of those experiencing such strokes died of them, and less than 20 percent had any further little stroke episodes, report Drs. S. G. Leonberg, Jr., and Frank A. Elliott.   (N-27)

CHAPTER 14

Obstetrics and Gynecology

A better time for conception?

Can the timing of conception have any significant influence on the likelihood of successful pregnancy?

Evidence suggesting that it can comes from a study in Colombia, South America, in which the rate of miscarriage, or spontaneous abortion, was linked to when the coitus responsible for conception took place in relation to ovulation, or release of the ovum.

Basal body temperature is a reliable test for ovulation. The fact that a rise of a few tenths of a degree in the temperature occurs one or two days before release of an ovum from an ovary is routinely used in family planning clinics employing the rhythm method and in sterility clinics. Such clinics also commonly keep records of coitus.

Records of coitus and ovulation for 965 women were obtained from clinics in Colombia, the United States, Canada, and France by Dr. Rodrigo Guerrero, an American-trained physician, now at the Department of Preventive Medicine of the Universidad del Vallas Medical School in Cali, Colombia, and a colleague, Dr. Ocar I. Rojas.

Of the 965 women, seventy-five miscarried, and the investigators could analyze the circumstances.

Although the overall miscarriage rate was 7.8 percent, there was a wide range of miscarriage probability—all the way from a peak of 24 percent, twenty-four chances out of one hundred, when insemination took place three days after the temperature shift, to a low of 3.2 percent when it took place two days before the shift.

Apparently, what had been found to be true in many animal studies—a higher probability of miscarriage associated with aging of ova or spermatazoa—held for humans.

Conceptions resulting from insemination on days two and three after the rise in temperature would be more likely to result from aged ova that had to wait for the sperm. And conceptions resulting from insemination three, four, and more days before the temperature shift probably resulted from aged sperm that had to wait for release of the ovum.

The study, indeed, showed probabilities of miscarriage highest at both extremes: 11.1 percent on the ninth day before the temperature shift; 7.1 percent on the eighth day; 19.3 percent on the seventh day; 7.3 percent on the sixth; 10.6 percent on the fifth, and 11.8 percent on the fourth; and, at the other extreme, 9.1 percent on the second day after the shift, and 24 percent on the third day.

In the middle—from day three before the shift to day one afterward—miscarriage probabilities were lowest: 5.5 percent for day three before; 3.2 percent for day two before; 7 percent for day one before; 7.5 percent for the day of the shift; and 5.5 percent for the first day afterward.

Thus the study suggests that coitus intended to lead to conception—if it takes place in the middle time period when both spermatazoa and ovum are likely to be freshest—is most likely to result in a successful pregnancy.   (OB-1)

When bleeding occurs early in pregnancy

It does in a sizeable proportion of women, and the outlook is not nearly as grim as once thought to be the case.

Studying a series of 6,223 pregnancies, University of California, Berkeley, and Kaiser Foundation Research Institute, Oakland, California, investigators found that 1,200 of the women experienced uterine bleeding—most frequently between the fourth and seventh weeks of pregnancy.

In some women, the bleeding was followed by almost immediate loss of the fetus. In 941 of the women, however, pregnancy continued and in more than three-fourths resulted in normal delivery at term.   (OB-2)

Miscarriage and excessive coffee consumption

Any or several of many factors may contribute to reproduction difficulties. Research has shown that excessive drinking and smoking may have detrimental effects on an unborn fetus.

That excessive coffee intake may also have such effects is indicated by data, which still have to be regarded as preliminary and far from definitive, from a study by Drs. Paul Weathersbee, J. R. Lodge, and L. K. Olsen of the University of Illinois at Urbana-Champaign.

Specifically, the study suggests that pregnant women who drink more than half a dozen cups of coffee a day may be increasing chances of miscarriage.

Of 550 women checked, fourteen said that they drank an average of seven cups or more daily. Thirteen of the fourteen had unfavorable pregnancies.

Caffeine, the investigators note, is one of the substances that can pass through the placenta from mother to fetus, and recent research indicates that fetuses may not be able to metabolize or break down the caffeine. When it is not properly metabolized, the caffeine appears to have a damaging effect on cells.   (OB-3)

A promising finding for habitual miscarriers

Veterinarians have known that certain organisms, called T-strain mycoplasma, can cause infertility in animals. But there was no suspicion of any possible effect in pregnant women until Dr. Ruth B. Kundsin, a bacteriologist at Peter Bent Brigham Hospital, Boston, isolated the organisms from miscarried human fetuses.

Recently, at Boston Hospital for Women, Dr. Herbert W. Horne, Jr., a gynecologist specializing in fertility problems, has been looking for mycoplasma in patients with those problems and treating the organisms when discovered.

The results of treatment are promising. Where, in his first twenty years of coping with infertility, he has reported, the miscarriage rate among successful conceptions was 20 percent, effective mycoplasma treatment has halved that figure.

Transmitted sexually, mycoplasma can live for years in the male or female genital tract. Often they produce no symptoms. In some women, they cause vaginitis (inflammation of the vagina), cervicitis (inflammation of the cervix), or recurrent cystitis (bladder inflammation).

To detect mycoplasma infection, a urine sample and samples from the cervical mucus are collected, placed in a culture to grow the organisms if they are present, sent to a laboratory, and checked at three days and again at one week.

Because culturing is relatively difficult and expensive, Dr. Horne and his associates use certain criteria to determine which women should be tested for mycoplasma—those with cervicitis, recurrent cystitis, previous histories of miscarriage, among them.

When the test is positive, both husband and wife are treated with a 10-day course of demeclocycline hydrochloride, an antibiotic effective against mycoplasma. In most cases, the medication causes little or no discomfort, but about 20 percent of patients experience nausea, vomiting, diarrhea, or urinary problems severe enough to require cessation of treatment.   (OB-4)

A drug to stop premature labor

When premature uterine contractions develop, a drug called indomethacin often may be helpful, according to a report from Israel. Indomethacin has been used previously for an entirely different purpose—to help relieve the discomfort of arthritis.

Physicians at the Central Emek Hospital, Afula, Israel, headed by Dr. H. Zuckerman, report that in 76 percent of a group of 98 women with premature contractions, the drug led to cessation of labor for periods of one to twelve weeks and seventy-five babies were born at maturity.   (OB-5)

Overdue babies

More and more physicians recently have come to consider it advisable not to allow babies to be more than two weeks overdue because of increased risk of death.

Other reasons as well for inducing birth soon after the due date are suggested by a study of 116 babies born fourteen or more days late, carried out by Dr. Keith Lovell of Queen Victoria Hospital, Adelaide, Australia.

Compared with on-time babies, Lovell found, twice as many of the overdue (14.7 percent) had to be delivered by cesarean section. The overdue infants also had a somewhat greater risk of breathing difficulty at birth and greater tendency to lose weight.

The study, Dr. Lovell reports, indicates that induction of birth, when necessary, between the fortieth and forty-second week, increases the likelihood of easier birth and healthier baby.   (OB-6)

Diabetic pregnancies

Diabetes carries a higher risk of intrauterine fetal death. But the risk can be decreased and the likelihood of delivery of a live, healthy baby increased greatly with effective control of the blood-sugar level.

Striking evidence of this has come from a ten-year Swedish study of diabetic pregnancies.

At Sahlgren's Hospital, Göteborg, physicians found a mortality rate of 23.6 percent for the babies of mothers with a mean blood-sugar level above 150 milligrams per 100 milliliters. The death rate fell to 13 percent in those with sugar levels of 100 to 150 milligrams per 100 milliliters, and to 3.8 percent in those with mean levels below 100 milligrams. A decreased morbidity or sickness rate in the infants accompanied the increased survival rate.   (OB-7)

Smoking and pregnancy

Two recent studies—one in Canada, the other in England—offer data on the influence of maternal cigarette smoking during pregnancy on the health and development of the child.

The study in Quebec involved a 10 percent random sample of 1970 and 1971 births and found that smoking substantially reduced average birth weight and increased by 24 percent the risk of death for the baby at or soon after birth.

The National Child Development Study in England, which has followed fifteen hundred children from birth through age eleven years, indicates that children of mothers who smoked ten or more cigarettes a day are, years after birth, on the average about one-fifth of an inch shorter and three to five months retarded in reading, mathematics, and general ability compared with children of nonsmoking mothers.   (OB-8)

Aspirin in pregnancy

Aspirin is so commonly used that it often is not even considered to be a drug. As well as other people, pregnant women use it and many use it frequently. One study at a Houston, Texas, hospital found that 60 percent of pregnant women used an analgesic, or pain reliever, at least several times a week and about 40 percent used an analgesic specifically containing aspirin.

A recent Australian study suggests that it may be wise to use the drug with caution during pregnancy.

The study, by physicians at the Royal Alexandra Hospital for Children in Sidney, compared 144 aspirin-using women with nonusers. The aspirin-users were divided into two groups: Group One, consisting of sixty-three women who used analgesics every day during pregnancy; Group Two, eighty-one women using analgesics at least once a week.

All the regular aspirin users, but especially those in Group One using it daily, experienced more problems than nonusers.

Women in Group One were twice as likely as nonusers to have anemia. The daily users had a significant mean increase in pregnancy duration—two weeks—and four times as many had pregnancies lasting longer than forty-two weeks. Their duration of labor was somewhat longer—5.6 hours versus 4.8 for nonusers—and their delivery complication rate three times as great.

Group One women had a stillbirth rate of eight in 150 pregnancies; Group Two, four in 128; the non-users, three in 200.   (OB-9)

Seat belts and pregnancy

The combination of automobile seat belt plus shoulder harness, not seat belt alone, provides maximum protection for the unborn child, according to a study with animals.

At the University of Oklahoma Health Sciences Center, Oklahoma City, a team headed by Dr. W. M. Crosby subjected twenty-two pregnant baboons to impacts comparable to those occurring in car accidents. The fetal death rate was 50 percent with seat belt alone, 8.34 percent with combination of belt and shoulder harness, and the high rate with belt alone appeared to be due not to sudden stop alone but to forward bending over the belt, preventable with shoulder harness.   (OB-10)

The right weight BEFORE pregnancy

Achieving proper weight before a child is conceived—either by reducing weight or gaining it if necessary—statistically increases the likelihood of having a healthy baby, according to a study of 87,858 births at twenty-two hospitals carried out by Dr. Istvan Nyirjesy of Georgetown University Medical Center, Washington, D.C.

The study found that risk of having a dangerously small baby or an infant dying just prior to or shortly after birth is least for a woman of average weight prior to becoming pregnant. (Because few women are short enough to weigh under 110 pounds and few tall enough to weigh more than 150, 110 to 150 is the range of average weight.)

In the investigation, women weighing less than 110 prior to pregnancy had a significantly higher percentage of children weighing under five and a half pounds at birth, stillborn, or dying within the first twenty-eight days after birth. Women with prepregnancy weights over 150 were not as likely to have small babies but they, too, had higher risk than normal-weight women of having stillborn babies and infants dying within the first twenty-eight days after birth.

In his own practice, since carrying out the study, Nyirjesy reports, he has been urging women to get to proper weight before becoming pregnant, postponing pregnancy for several months if necessary in order to do so. (OB-11)

Maternal infections and pregnancy outcome

Surprising findings come from a study of four hundred women who, during pregnancy, contracted either measles, mumps, chickenpox, or hepatitis.

Although many physicians as well as lay people have believed that any such infection increases the likelihood of malformation for the baby, the study found no such increase. While 2.2 percent of the infants had defects at birth, the proportion was about the same as for infants of mothers who had not been infected.

But some undesirable effects of infection were noted. Hepatitis in the last half of pregnancy did increase risk of premature birth and early infant mortality. Measles seemed to increase the prematurity rate. Mumps in the first three months of pregnancy led to an increase in miscarriage. (OB-12)

Pyelonephritis in pregnancy

Acute pyelonephritis, or kidney inflammation, occurs in 1.3 percent of all pregnancies. In addition to producing high temperature, malaise, and back and flank pain, often requiring hospitalization, the infection is often associated with premature labor.

Antibiotic treatment is usually effective for the immediate attack but recurrences are frequent. A recent study indicates how the rate of recurrence can be drastically reduced.

At Wilford Hall USAF Medical Center, Lackland Air Force Base, San Antonio, women with acute pyelonephritis were divided into two groups. Those in one group received the usual antibiotic treatment during the acute episode and for two weeks afterward. For women in the second group, antibiotic therapy was continued for the rest of pregnancy.

Sixty percent of the patients in the first group had recurrences requiring hospitalization. Only 2.7 percent of those receiving continued treatment had a recurrence. (OB-13)

A vitamin to suppress milk flow

For women who do not breast-feed, lactation, or milk secretion, is suppressed by application of ice bags and a tight binder to the breasts after delivery. The breasts usually become painfully engorged for two or three days and analgesics may be needed. Some physicians use an estrogen preparation for several days.

Vitamin B_6, according to a recent British study, appears to be particularly effective for lactation suppression.

In the investigation with 254 women, 95 percent of those receiving a 200-milligram tablet of the vitamin three times a day as compared to 83 percent of those receiving an estrogen preparation had milk secretion suppressed within one week.

The speed with which symptoms were relieved also differed: ten hours for B_6, more than twenty-four hours for the estrogen preparation. (OB-14)

The value—and neglect—of prenatal diagnosis

Prenatal diagnosis—using a test, amniocentesis (described below)—can be increasingly valuable in detecting the presence, and no less important, the absence, of genetic disorders in the fetus. Yet it is greatly underused.

Genetic disorders constitute a vast, often tragic burden. It is estimated that total life-years lost from genetically caused birth defects is three and a half times that due to cancer, six and a half times that due to heart disease, and eight times that due to stroke. About 40 percent of all infant mortality is due to genetic disorders. Almost one-third of all pediatric patients and 10 percent of all adult patients require hospitalization because of genetic disorders. Yet currently only about two thousand women a year are undergoing prenatal diagnostic testing.

The procedure. Amniocentesis, usually carried out during the fifteenth or sixteenth week of pregnancy, involves taking a small sample of the fluid surrounding the fetus by means of a hollow needle passed through the mother's abdomen into the womb. The fluid contains castoff fetal cells which can be analyzed for signs of disorders. The test can be carried out by any experienced obstetrician on an outpatient basis.

The capability. Through amniocentesis, the sex of the child can be determined, and that is valuable for sex-linked disorders such as hemophilia and Duchenne's muscular dystrophy, which affect only males, although females may be carriers.

Amniocentesis can reveal Down's syndrome (mongolism), which occurs in one of every seven hundred births. And it is capable of detecting a steadily increasing list of genetic disorders, including Fabry's disease (with kidney failure and death in young adulthood), Lesch-Nyhan syndrome (with severe mental and physical retardation), Hunter's syndrome (often producing death in the first decade), disorders of fat metabolism that often lead to death in early childhood, Tay-Sachs disease, Saddhoff's disease, and maple syrup urine disease, also often fatal, and still others.

Accuracy and safety. Amniocentesis is remarkably accurate— better than 99 percent predictive, according to a Northwestern University study with seven hundred women.

The safety is high, as demonstrated by a recently completed government study which compared the experience of 1,040 women who had amniocentesis with a matched group of other pregnant women who did not receive the test. There were no significant differences between the two groups in rates of miscarriage, stillbirth, maternal complications, prematurity, fetal injury, or other untoward effects.

At one year of age, the two sets of infants showed no significant difference in growth and development.

The several values. One value of prenatal diagnosis is obvious. It can detect in the fetal stage thousands who, if permitted to be born, would die early in life and many others who would suffer from varying degrees of mental retardation and from complications due to defects of vital organs or body systems. It can eliminate much suffering by giving parents of a fetus virtually certain to be born seriously defective the alternative of abortion, and the opportunity to try again with the chance, often great, of a better outcome.

Also, in at least a few cases now and undoubtedly more in the future, detection of a genetic problem may be followed by treatment for it while the fetus is still in the womb.

One of the first successes in treatment has been achieved with an inherited disorder, methylmalonic acidemia, in which acids accumulate abnormally in the body, leading to recurrent vomiting, developmental retardation and failure to thrive, and death.

The case involved a Boston woman whose first child had been born with methylmalonic acidemia and had died at three months. Amniocentesis in her second pregnancy revealed the same problem again.

Vitamin B_{12} is an essential for normal handling of materials in the body if methylmalonic acid buildup is to be avoided. The fetus was not producing enough of the vitamin. Pediatricians at Tufts-New England Medical Center, Boston, decided to try giving the mother large doses of the vitamin in the hope that in that way enough could reach the baby to compensate for the deficiency. The baby was normal at birth and remains so eighteen months later.

Hardly the least of the values of prenatal diagnosis are the reassurance and encouragement it offers for many worried couples.

In more than 95 percent of cases, amniocentesis for diagnosis of possible defects discloses that the suspected defects are not present.

Of the 1,040 women who had amniocentesis in the previously mentioned government study, 995, or 95.7 percent, learned that their babies were not at risk. Another study by the National Foundation-March of Dimes found that of 2,187 women undergoing the procedure in 1974, 2,125, or 97.2 percent, learned that a suspected defect happily was not present.

In the opinion of many authorities, amniocentesis has great lifesaving value; without the definitive answer it provides, many couples, on the basis of only the statistical odds, opt for abortion.

Prenatal diagnosis for whom. Three categories of pregnant women can benefit from amniocentesis. One consists of women who already have borne a defective child. A second includes those who themselves have family history of a defect or whose husbands do. The third category consists of women over the age of about thirty-five for whom risks of bearing a defective child are increased.

Why underutilization. Since 1969, the state of Massachusetts has paid for amniocentesis analyses performed by the Genetics Laboratory at the Eunice Kennedy Shriver Center in Waltham, and obstetricians throughout the state have known about the program and the opportunity to send an amniocentesis sample to the laboratory for free analysis. But only 350 analyses per year have been done, representing a small fraction of women at risk in the state.

In Illinois, the laboratory at the Children's Memorial Hospital, Chicago, carries out 85 percent to 90 percent of all analyses in the state but has been doing only about one hundred a year. And the hospital's chief of staff notes that many of the patients, moreover, aren't referred by their physicians but come after learning about their risk and about the laboratory from the press and other sources. Clearly, he observes, doctors have been holding back.

To some extent, this may be because in medicine as in other areas there is always to be found some resistance to new developments. Until recently, too, there may have been some concern with safety of amniocentesis, but safety is now a well-documented fact.

Some physicians also may fail to recommend amniocentesis out of religious opposition to any abortion that may result. They are being urged now by such pioneers in the field as Drs. Cecil Jacobson of George Washington University and Michale M. Kaback of the University of California at Los Angeles to stop thinking of prenatal diagnosis solely in terms of abortion and start thinking of all the normal babies who could be delivered to women who might otherwise not dare to become pregnant after an initial catastrophe.   (OB-15)

Treatments for infertility

Inability to have children can stem from many possible causes. These are recently reported developments in the treatment of infertility.

Surgery for endometriosis. One cause of infertility is endometriosis, the presence of the endometrium, the tissue that lines the uterus, in sites where it does not belong such as the external surface of the uterus, in the ovary, or in the bladder or intestine.

After surgery to remove the tissue from abnormal sites, a medical team at Johns Hopkins University, Baltimore, has reported, fifty-two of 101 previously infertile women conceived, in most cases within the first year.   (OB-16)

Prolactin. A hormone secreted by the pituitary gland at the base of the brain, prolactin has long been known to promote the growth of breast tissue and stimulate milk production. Japanese physicians have reported that in some cases it may be an effective treatment for infertility.

At Kyushu University, Dr. Yasushi Okamura and associates have reported trying the hormone in fifteen women, all infertile for more than five years. Seven became pregnant. The women, aged twenty-five to thirty-six, received 100 to 200 international units of prolactin by intramuscular injection for several days around the time of ovulation. Five conceived during the first cycle after treatment began, and two during the second and third cycles.   (OB-17)

One clinic's findings. At a clinic for infertility problems run by the Jefferson Medical College, Philadelphia Division of Endocrinology, 1,236 couples with infertility problems were seen in a three-year period and 734, or approximately 60 percent, conceived.

The majority—795—were primary infertility cases, i.e., they had never had a conception in marriage. For 318 couples, there had been repeated miscarriage problems; infertility after having one child was the problem for 123 couples.

Because of the endocrine (gland) focus of the clinic, the great majority of patients seen had ovulatory defect problems.

In some cases, in the clinic's experience, reassurance alone, without treatment of any kind, resulted in conception after the first visit. In other cases, small doses of estrogen used in one phase of the menstrual cycle to enhance release of other hormones, gonadotropins, needed for ovulation helped. In still others, human menopausal gonadotropins (Pergonal) were of benefit.

When these measures failed, an ovulation-inducing agent such as clomiphene citrate often was of value. The latter sometimes leads to multiple births, and five twin births occurred.

In only twelve cases did premature labor occur. There were sixty-seven cases of miscarriage, mostly in women who had habitually miscarried before.

All told, among those seeking help because of the miscarriage problem, the success rate was 73 percent; among those in the primary and one-child infertility groups who conceived, almost 90 percent successfully gave birth to a child.   (OB-18)

Does adoption help? A common belief is that adoption of a child by an infertile couple may improve the likelihood that they will conceive one of their own. But a study at the Infertility Center of the Royal Victorian Hospital and McGill University, Montreal, fails to bear out the belief.

In the study, 533 infertile couples were followed until conception or for five years. A child was adopted by 133 couples; 20 percent thereafter conceived a child of their own. Among the couples who did not adopt, the conception rate was 66 percent.   (OB-19)

Hypnosis for infertility? Apparently, in some cases, hypnosis may have some usefulness, in the admittedly very limited experience of an Ottawa physician, Dr. E. Napke.

His first experience was with a woman infertile for six years for whom hypnosis was being used for another problem. She became pregnant, now has four children.

In a second case, a course of hypnosis was followed by pregnancy in a woman infertile for four years.

A third woman, also infertile for an extended period, could not be hypnotized.

In the fourth case reported by Dr. Napke, a woman with failure of menstruation and infertility, who had not responded to hormone treatment, became pregnant four months after starting hypnosis and gave birth to a healthy girl.   (OB-20)

Varicocele and male infertility. Varicocele—a varicose condition of the veins of the spermatic cord—appears to be a relatively common cause of infertility in men. In a five-year study, Drs. Lawrence Dubin and Richard Amelar of New York University School of Medicine found varicocele to be at fault in 39 percent of more than twelve hundred infertile men.

The problem can be corrected readily by surgery. In 80 percent of men operated on, semen quality improved and 48 percent of wives became pregnant, Drs. Dubin and Amelar reported.

More recently, the same two investigators reported additional experience with 540 subfertile men who underwent varicocele correction. Overall, semen quality improved in 71 percent and 55 percent of wives became pregnant.

Results proved to be best in men with preoperative sperm counts of 10 million per milliliter, with 88 percent showing improved counts and 68 percent of wives becoming pregnant. In those with lower preoperative sperm counts, 33 percent showed improvement and 23 percent of wives became pregnant. For this latter group, a trial after surgery of human chorionic gonadotropin, a hormone found in pregnancy urine, improved sperm counts in 56 percent and increased the pregnancy rate to 44 percent.   (OB-21)

Clomiphene for men. Clomiphene citrate, the fertility drug that has sometimes been too successful in infertile women, leading to multiple-birth pregnancies, may have some usefulness in some men.

In a trial at Duke University School of Medicine, Durham, North Carolina, Drs. David F. Paulson and Jeff Wacksman gave the drug for twenty-five days each month for up to six months to twenty-two men with abnormally low sperm counts. In nineteen, the counts rose toward normal.

Best results were obtained in thirteen men whose sperm counts to begin with were thirty million per cubic centimeter or higher. In all thirteen, sperm counts rose toward and, in some cases, exceeded normal fertility levels of 120 million, with pregnancies occurring, at the time of the report, in three wives.   (OB-22)

Mycoplasma and male infertility. Male infertility can be complex, not always easy to diagnose since there are many possible causes, including physical obstructions to the passage of sperm, hormonal imbalances, injuries, drugs, psychological disturbances, and still others.

One of the "still others," it now appears, may be T mycoplasma organisms which have also been found to be involved in some women who miscarry (see "A promising finding for habitual miscarriers," page 00).

At the University of Uppsala in Sweden, Drs. Hakan Gnarpe and Jan Friberg isolated the organisms from the semen of men with unexplained infertility. Suspecting that the organisms might have something to do with the infertility, they gave the men antibiotic treatment. Afterward, the wives of 30 percent of the men became pregnant. Using the extremely high-powered scanning electron microscope, the investigators were able to determine that the organisms actually attach themselves to the sperm cells of men with reproductive failure.   (OB-23)

Sterilization: increasingly simplified

Sterilization for women has become a relatively simple, quick procedure.

Less than five years ago, a report from the Chicago Lying-in Hospital noted successful results in 270 women with a ten-minute procedure for cutting and cauterizing the fallopian tubes performed under general anesthesia.

Through a small incision, little more than half an inch long, below the navel, a viewing instrument was inserted; through a second small incision, the tubes were cut and cauterized with another instrument; after which both incisions were closed and covered with adhesive strips. Only one day of hospitalization was required.   (OB-24)

More recently, doctors at Deaconess Hospital, Buffalo, New York, reported using much the same procedure in 1,020 women. In only fourteen was there any complication such as bleeding. And where at first one day of hospitalization was thought necessary, the procedure soon was being carried out on an outpatient basis with hospital stay cut to nine hours or less.   (OB-25)

Still more recently, a newer technique carried out under local anesthesia in ten to fifteen minutes has been developed by Dr. InBae Yoon of Johns Hopkins Hospital, Baltimore, and used successfully in hundreds of women there and elsewhere.

It requires only a small incision in the abdomen to allow each fallopian tube to be drawn into a loop that is then held securely and permanently by a silicone rubber ring. Patients go home a few hours later.   (OB-26)

Abortion: safest time, safest kind

A study of abortions carried out in New York City after legalization of abortion has found that more than two-thirds of those being obtained legally would otherwise have been obtained illegally.

The study also indicated that legal, expertly performed abortions are remarkably safe, especially when carried out during the first three months of pregnancy. The death rate of 1.7 per 100,000 is lower than the maternal death rate of fourteen per 100,000 in childbirth, even lower than the mortality rate of five per 100,000 for tonsillectomy/ adenoidectomy. Abortions during the second three months of pregnancy do carry a higher risk of 12.2 deaths per 100,000.   (OB-27)

Another study in New York City of 402,000 women having legal abortions in a two-year period determined that the safest abortion technique is vacuum aspiration or suction; next safest is dilatation and curettage; and third safest is introduction of saline solution. (OB-28)

For cystic disease of the breast: an oral contraceptive

One of the most common breast disorders, cystic disease, a benign condition, may give the breast a "cobblestone" feel and produce pain or premenstrual discomfort.

Surgery—simple excision of the diseased area—may be used. But periodic medical observation with aspiration of larger cysts may be all that is needed since the condition tends to improve following menopause.

Recently, use of an oral contraceptive, norethynodrel with mestranol (Enovid), has been reported by Dr. I. M. Ariel of the Pack Medical Group, New York City. On an average dose of 5 milligrams three times a day, seventy-six of 110 women showed improvement in the disease itself and sixty-eight had relief of pain or discomfort. The most frequent side effect was weight gain which could be checked by use of a diuretic drug.   (OB-29)

Breast lump: a quick, anxiety-relieving test

Between the time a lump in a breast is first discovered and the time a small section of it is removed under general anesthesia in a hospital for microscopic study can be a period of acute anxiety.

Much of the anxiety may be avoided by a simple aspiration test that permits determination within an hour whether the lump is benign or malignant, report Drs. Tilde S. Kline and Hunter S. Neal of Lankenau Hospital, Philadelphia.

For the test, a needle is inserted into a suspect lump, suction is applied, and a tissue sample quickly withdrawn.

In a trial at the hospital, 273 of 324 lumps checked proved to be benign. In fifteen of the remainder, with further testing, an indication of abnormality was found to be erroneous.

The aspiration test accurately indicated malignancy in thirty of thirty-six cancerous lumps, including three missed by mammography.   (OB-30)

Help for vaginitis

Vaginitis, or vaginal inflammation, is a common problem, affecting at any one time as many as one-third of all women of childbearing age. In addition, it can affect very young girls and older women.

Most forms of vaginitis are caused by overgrowth of microorganisms normally present in small numbers in the vagina without producing ill effects.

A most common, troublesome type is candidiasis, caused by a fungus resembling yeast. The most common symptom is intense itching. A discharge, usually described as white and "cheesy," may or may not be present.

Although an antifungal drug, candicidin, is helpful, recurrences after its use are frequent. The drug is usually taken in tablet form.

Its use in ointment form instead may produce superior results, according to a study by Dr. Kenneth Morese of Good Samaritan Hospital, Suffern, New York. Admittedly, Dr. Morese notes, tablets are less messy to use but it is the messiness of the ointment that apparently leads to better distribution of the drug and a higher cure rate.

Only three of forty-nine women using the ointment for a two-week period as against twelve of fifty-one using tablets required a second course of treatment for relief of symptoms. And long-term follow-up has shown recurrences in almost twice as many in the tablet-treated, eleven patients, as in the ointment-treated, six patients.   (OB-31)

It also appears now that boric acid, when properly prescribed by a physician, can be a safe, effective, and inexpensive treatment for candidiasis.

Drs. T. E. Swate and J. C. Weed of the Ochsner Clinic and Foundation Hospital, New Orleans, report first determining in laboratory studies that boric acid stops the growth of the fungus, then employing it for forty patients, all of whom were relieved of symptoms. A follow-up at thirty days after treatment showed thirty-eight of the forty free of recurrence.   (OB-32)

Douching: is it really essential?

Although commonly believed to be, it is not necessary for normal or routine feminine hygiene, according to a recent report, which adds that many women can live a lifetime in good health without douching.

The vagina has a normal microorganism population completely compatible with good health, and there is no evidence that the incidence of vaginal and uterine infections is reduced by regular douching.

No harm will be done if a woman chooses to use vaginal lavage in moderation—two to four times a month—but daily douching is to be discouraged. Any commercial douche preparation or a simple mixture of one ounce of white vinegar in one quart of water is adequate, the report notes.   (OB-33)

Treating urinary tract infection

Chronic urinary tract infection related to sexual intercourse is not uncommon in women. In the experience of Dr. Kenneth L. Vosti of the Stanford University School of Medicine, short-term medical treatment for flare-ups of infection has not prevented recurrences. Nor, in many cases, have such practices, although often advised by physicians, as scrubbing the perineum before coitus and emptying the bladder afterward.

So, in a trial, Dr. Vosti had fourteen patients with chronic urinary infection give themselves a dose of antibiotic—penicillin G, nitrofurantoin, cephalexin, nalidixic acid, or a sulfonamide—after sexual intercourse for nineteen to 111 months each, or a total of 761 months.

During those 761 months, the women experienced a total of nineteen infections—significantly fewer than the ninety infections recorded during 705 previous months when they were not taking preventive antibiotics.   (OB-34)

New treatments for genital herpes

Caused by the same herpes simplex virus responsible for cold sores and fever blisters, genital herpes, also known as herpes genitalis, can produce painful, persistent, and in some women frequently recurring, vaginal sores, with pain becoming almost unbearable in some cases during urination.

When a topical anesthetic, such as lidocaine ointment, fails to provide relief for the painful urination, Dr. Te-Wen Chang of Tufts-

New England Medical Center has found that a simple measure will provide relief and it can be carried out in any restroom.

A small plastic bottle with spray top is filled with cold water. When the water is sprayed onto the painful area immediately upon start of urination and repeatedly during the process it eliminates the pain throughout.   (OB-35)

A dye/light treatment for herpes genitalis. At the Baylor College of Medicine, Houston, a medical team headed by Dr. Raymond H. Kaufman have obtained promising results with a treatment that involves painting the vaginal sores with a dye, 0.1% proflavine, then exposing the area to either fluorescent light or 150 watts of incandescent light from a six-inch distance for ten minutes, repeating the procedure immediately, and then again twenty-four hours later. Of the first forty-nine women so treated, twenty-three had immediate pain relief and sixteen others experienced relief within two days.   (OB-36)

Vaccine treatment. BCG, a vaccine originally developed for use against tuberculosis, has a stimulating effect on the body's immune system, helping it to resist infection. BCG also has been used with some promise to stimulate the immune system as an aid in combatting some cancers.

A small-scale early study suggests that BCG may have value against herpes genitalis. In all of fifteen women receiving it, there has been a significant fall in the frequency of recurrent infections. (OB-37)

Cystitis and tub-bathing

Cystitis, or bladder infection, is a recurrent problem for many women. Infection may be eliminated successfully enough by extended antibiotic treatment (four weeks or more), only to return.

On a hunch that tub-bathing might possibly have something to do with reinfection, one investigator, Dr. Robert S. Gould of Wellesley, Massachusetts, prescribed showers instead of tub baths for fifty women who had had multiple recurrences (as many as ten). As long as they avoided the baths, thirty-four remained free of infection. Twelve of the sixteen who developed recurrent infections had resumed baths.

Following the original study, Dr. Gould reports, of five hundred women with cystitis, only three failed to benefit from at least one month of antibiotic treatment coupled with bath avoidance. (OB-38)

A simple operation for urinary incontinence

In a procedure developed by Dr. Thomas Stamey of Stanford University School of Medicine, control often can be restored for women troubled with urinary incontinence without need for major abdominal or pelvic surgery.

The urinary bladder is simply tightened with a suture on either side, placed accurately with specially designed needles. The procedure is carried out through a cystoscope, the same instrument used for diagnostic examination.

Ninety percent of women undergoing the procedure, Dr. Stamey reports, have experienced marked improvement or been completely cured of incontinence.   (OB-39)

CHAPTER 15

Pediatrics

Passive babies, bright future

Some newborns seemingly passive early in life—breathing slowly, relatively insensitive to touch, responding lethargically even to interruption of sucking—cause parents worry that they are backward children.

Yet just such infants are apt to mature into intelligent, responsive youngsters, according to a study by Dr. Richard Q. Bell and other investigators at the National Institute of Mental Health, Bethesda, Maryland. In the study, the children's development was checked from infancy up through seven and one-half years of age.

One possible explanation offered for why the early passive later tend to outdo the early more responsive and vigorous babies is that overly aroused and responsive infants may in some fashion adversely affect parental behavior toward them, making them less likely to develop as assertive, sociable, enthusiastic youngsters. Conceivably, too, if an infant is vigorous, restless, and irritable, so much of a mother's time may go into caretaking that little is left for healthy social interaction with the child.   (P-1)

The rhythmic babies

Although there has been some notion that infants who rhythmically rock their bodies, roll their heads, or kick their legs may be emotionally disturbed, they are, in fact, quite normal, according to a twelve-year study of rhythmic habit patterns carried out by Dr. Harvey Kravitz of Children's Memorial Hospital, Chicago.

Normal, healthy children, Kravitz reports, commonly exhibit rhythmic patterns, even of hand sucking, soon after birth and develop more rhythmic patterns as they grow older, a sign that they are learning new skills and their nervous systems are developing. In contrast, low-birth-weight children and those with breathing difficulties or other problems often take longer to develop rhythmic patterns. Urges Kravitz: Allow a baby to kick, bang, rock, and the like as much as he wishes; he is likely to be developing normally.   (P-2)

Better feeding for "preemies"

To bring about weight gain in premature and other low-birth-weight infants, feeding formula through a tube passed into the stomach often has been required. But that has caused problems of overfilling tiny stomachs, leading sometimes to regurgitation and breathing difficulties.

Now those problems have been avoided and better results obtained by using a nonirritating plastic tube that can be passed beyond the stomach into the intestine.

At Michael Reese Medical Center, Chicago, Dr. John B. Paton and other physicians report that with the new technique, used successfully on 250 infants, birth weight is regained in five to seven days, half the time needed with stomach feeding.   (P-3)

Iron for babies

Infants require iron to avoid iron-deficiency anemia. Iron-supplemented infant cereals are available but, in themselves, do not provide enough iron, whereas iron-supplemented formulas do, according to a study with seventy babies, aged four to seven months, by Dr. Ernesto Rios and other physicians of the University of Washington, Seattle.

The study determined that not more than 1 percent of iron compounds in cereals is absorbed; but the average 4.2 percent absorption rate from iron-fortified formulas is adequate.   (P-4)

Treating congenital hip dislocation

A small proportion of infants are born with hip instability which may lead to hip dislocation. The instability was found in thirty of 3,278 consecutive newborns examined by Dr. M. A. Ritter of Indiana University School of Medicine, Indianapolis.

The thirty affected infants were treated with an aluminum malleable brace worn continuously for six weeks. Once the hip became stable, brace and all restrictions were eliminated. Checked again by physical examination and X-ray study three months and then one year later, all but one of the thirty proved to be normal.   (P-5)

Head tilting attacks

Its cause not clear, paroxysmal torticollis produces episodes during which a baby keeps his head tilted to one side. Studying twelve children with the problem, Dr. C. H. Snyder of the Ochsner Clinic, New Orleans, found that the attacks usually began between the ages of two and eight months, lasted two to three days at a time, and recurred two to three times a month. In seven of the twelve children, vomiting and pallor accompanied the episodes; the other five youngsters seemed unperturbed despite severe head tilt. No treatment was of any value but happily, Dr. Snyder found, the torticollis episodes usually disappear spontaneously around two to three years of age.
          (P-6)

Baby shoes: are special ones really needed?

Despite a common belief that they are as a means of promoting normal foot development and avoiding foot problems, a survey of 279 pediatricians shows that more than three-fourths consider inexpensive rubber-soled sneakers to be just as adequate as much higher-priced high-top leather shoes for infants with normal feet. Only about 20 percent of pediatricians believe that soft soles, high tops, and straight lasts are of particular value.

Noteworthy, too: an American Academy of Pediatrics-American Medical Association handbook remarks that a baby doesn't need shoes to learn to walk or for support unless a foot deformity is present. Shoes, it reports, are unnecessary until a child begins to walk and needs protection from hard surfaces—and then "any type of shoe that provides this protection will do." (P-7)

Shaking small babies—AVOID IT

An infant's head is relatively heavy, his neck muscles weak, his brain immature. And shaking a young child—as a well-meant disciplinary measure—can be extremely dangerous, causing whiplash brain damage, small but cumulative bleeding within head and eyes that can lead to cerebral palsy, mental retardation, vision impairment, or even death. So reports Dr. John Caffey of the University of Pittsburgh School of Medicine who has spent many years studying the problem. Shaking, he reports, is undoubtedly responsible for many of the cerebrovascular injuries attributed to prenatal infections, congenital malformations, birth injuries, and genetic metabolic diseases. "Infants, particularly infantile heads," he emphasizes, "should be handled and jolted as little as possible under all circumstances." (P-8)

Breathholding children

Understandably anxiety-provoking for parents, breathholding episodes in children are actually innocuous, Dr. Samuel Livingston of Johns Hopkins University School of Medicine has found after extensive studies.

Typically, the spells appear during the first two years of life but hardly ever before age six months. The pattern is fairly uniform: the child, after becoming angry or fearful, or after injuring himself even slightly, begins to cry, suddenly gasps, holds his breath, appears to be in a rage, almost always becomes blue, then rigid, and may suffer impaired consciousness. But unconsciousness is brief and harmless.

The spells tend to occur in families, almost exclusively in normally intelligent children, and produce no indications of brain damage, and the prognosis is excellent. No drugs are needed; none, in fact, are of value. But the spells usually can be counted on to disappear spontaneously after the age of four, Dr. Livingston finds.

Parents, he advises, should display an attitude of "purposeful neglect" so the child does not get any satisfaction from the breath-holding spells nor come to use them to dominate the family. Very much to be avoided: indulgence on the one hand, undue severity on the other, inconsistency. If this advice, says Dr. Livingston, is followed and combined with recognition that the attacks are rarely harmful to the child and the outlook good, most parents will cope well with the situation.   (P-9)

Bowlegs and knock-knees

At certain ages, both are virtually normal, need no treatment in otherwise healthy youngsters, and in most cases correct themselves, report Drs. L. A. Greenberg and A. A. Swartz of the University of Miami.

Most commonly, bowlegs appear between ages one and two, knock-knees between ages three and four. In some cases, bowlegs may progress to knock-knees and the progression occurred in nine of twenty-four untreated children and also in seven of twenty-eight whose bowlegs were corrected by treatment. Of thirty-six children with knock-knees who were studied, none showed a transition to bowlegs, and only two were treated orthopedically.

Based on their findings, the two doctors report, correction of either condition occurs spontaneously as often as when a child is treated.   (P-10)

Thumb-sucking

Almost half of children under four years of age—45.6 percent—suck their thumbs. And in a young child, the habit doesn't necessarily indicate emotional problems and need be of no concern.

If an infant sucks his thumb, suggests Dr. M. E. J. Curzon of the Eastman Dental Center, Rochester, New York, a mother would be well advised to determine that the baby is getting enough nursing to satisfy needs for oral gratification. If not, a pacifier can be used and is more readily abandoned, later, than thumb-sucking.

When a child under three sucks thumb or finger, ignoring the habit rather than calling attention to it is likely to lead to its being given up by age four. If it continues at four, especially if it is constant throughout the day, a dentist should be consulted for suggestions and, if necessary, for treatment to prevent malocclusion.   (P-11)

Swallowed objects

Coins, marbles, and such are often swallowed by children, lodge in the esophagus, and in the past have required hospitalization, general anesthesia, and use of an instrument, an esophagoscope, for removal.

A new removal technique, avoiding need for anesthesia and hospitalization, has been reported by Drs. G. D. Shackelford and W. H. McAlister of Washington University School of Medicine, Saint Louis, and Charles L. Robertson of Saint Luke's Hospital, Boise, Idaho.

A deflated balloon at the end of a small tube is passed through the nose and, while being viewed by fluoroscope, is slipped below the foreign object. The balloon is then inflated to expand the esophagus and the foreign object is pulled up ahead of the balloon. Without even need for sedation, the technique has allowed ready extraction not only of coins and marbles but plastic toys and even a small battery.   (P-12)

Repeated pain episodes in children

Recurrent episodes of abdominal or other pain occur in a surprising proportion of children, according to a study in which 18,162 observations among unselected children aged six to nineteen years were made.

Recurrent abdominal pain occurred in 14.4 percent, headache in 20.6 percent, limb (growing) pains in 15.5 percent. Abdominal pain proved to be most frequent at nine years, headache at twelve, and all types of pain occurred more often in girls than in boys.

All episodes also showed a tendency to disappear spontaneously

toward adulthood, although this was least true for girls'
headaches.   (P-13)

Abdominal epilepsy of childhood

Recurring attacks of abdominal pain (see above) are common in
children and commonly no usual cause can be found. But in some
cases, abdominal epilepsy—largely a childhood disorder and rare in
adults—may be responsible.

Typically, with abdominal epilepsy, there are attacks of mid- or
upper-abdominal pain lasting no more than a few minutes, sometimes
accompanied by nausea, vomiting, and appetite loss, and with some
confusion but no seizure or loss of consciousness. Usually, after an
episode, the child falls asleep and, upon awakening, feels well.

The vast majority of children with abdominal epilepsy, report Drs.
R. R. Babb and P. B. Eckman of the Palo Alto, California, Medical
Center, can be freed of symptoms with an anticonvulsive agent such
as diphenlhydantoin and, in fact, response to such a drug confirms the
diagnosis of abdominal epilepsy.   (P-14)

Treating bed-wetting children

In at least some persistent bed wetters, urinary tract allergy may be
responsible, and treatment for the allergy may end the problem.

Small bladder capacity is common in bed-wetting children and may
be the result of muscle spasm or contraction. In some, the spasm may
stem from allergy, report Drs. J. W. Gerrard and A. Zaleski of the
University of Saskatchewan, Saskatoon, Canada.

In a study in which twenty-five children were placed on a diet
excluding such common allergenic foods as cow's milk, dairy products, chocolate and cola drinks, eggs, citrus fruits and juices, and
tomatoes, five became completely continent and six others showed
marked improvement. In most of the remaining fourteen children,
imipramine, an antidepressant drug also commonly used for bed-
wetting, proved effective, and in all the youngsters improving on
either diet or drug, normal bladder capacity developed.   (P-15)

Help for osteogenesis imperfecta

Osteogenesis imperfecta is a disease in which bones, losing their normal complement of calcium, become porous and soft. Children with the disease not uncommonly suffer repeated arm and leg fractures, as many as a dozen a year, as the result of minor accidents. In addition, they may suffer from spinal curvature and remain small in stature.

Now a recently discovered thyroid hormone, calcitonin, is proving to be effective in arresting the disease. Children receiving the hormone, report Dr. Salvador Castells and a Downstate Medical Center, Brooklyn, New York, research team, have increased bone density, significantly reduced incidence of fractures, and achieved a spurt in growth.   (P-16)

Children with phenylketonuria (PKU)

PKU is a hereditary condition in which lack of an enzyme prevents proper body handling (metabolism) of an amino acid, phenylalanine, found in protein foods. The amino acid accumulates abnormally in blood and, if untreated, the condition leads to mental retardation and other manifestations such as tremors, poor muscular coordination, excessive perspiration, and in some cases convulsions.

The disorder can be detected at or shortly after birth by a simple test of the infant's urine—a test now required by law in some states. A special diet, begun in the first few weeks of life, allows the child to grow and develop normally. The diet is designed to restrict the intake of phenylalanine, and since few foods contain proteins lacking the amino acid, synthetic preparations of protein supplements are used.

Must the diet be used for a lifetime? A study suggesting that that may not be necessary has been carried out by Drs. William B. Hanley and Lydia Linsao of the University of Toronto with sixty-one young patients off the special diet for from one to five or more years.

Close follow-up of the children showed that since going off the diet forty-nine had experienced no change in IQ, seven showed an increase of up to twenty-three points, only five had a drop of more than ten points. No behavioral changes occurred in fifty-two of the youngsters, five showed improvement, only four deteriorated.

The study suggests that it is safe to take many, even most children

off the special diet at about the age of five, but all should be checked
medically from time to time so that, if necessary, the diet can be
resumed.   (P-17)

Children with poor appetites

Cyproheptadine, an antihistamine originally used for allergic skin
and other disorders, sometimes can be helpful in stimulating the
appetites of underdeveloped children, according to a study by Dr.
J. L. Penfold of the Hospital for Sick Children, Toronto.

Children receiving a three-month course of treatment with the
compound ate so well that their weight gain was some five times and
their growth about two times normal during the period.   (P-18)

Another hopeful development has been reported by Dr. K. M.
Hambidge and a University of Colorado Medical Center, Denver,
team. Zinc is a trace element found in minute amounts in many foods
and required by the body. Recently, in adults, taste disturbances and
even loss of taste have been found related to zinc deficiency and
improved with zinc therapy.

Zinc can be tested for in hair. The Denver physicians, testing
hundreds of subjects to determine zinc concentrations, discovered a
group of children with zinc levels of less than half found in others of
their age. Seventy percent of the low zinc children had a history of
poor appetite; 80 percent had inferior growth rates; 50 percent had
impaired taste sensations. In each child, small quantities of prescribed zinc increased the zinc levels in hair, led to normal taste
acuity, and may, it is hoped, lead to sustained improvement of both
appetite and growth rates.   (P-19)

Growth failure

A well-known reason for growth failure in children is lack of
adequate growth hormone from the pituitary gland at the base of the
brain. Another may be inadequate thyroid hormone secretion due to
hypothyroidism.

Levothyroxine, a thyroid preparation, may be of value in both
situations, according to a study at the National Pituitary Agency,
Baltimore, by Dr. Salvatore Raiti and colleagues. They followed
closely five children—two with pituitary insufficiency and three with

thyroid insufficiency—who received levothyroxine. The children grew three to five inches during the first year of thyroid treatment, and about two to three and one-half inches during the second year. (P-20)

When does growth stop?

Checking on the growth of almost two hundred children from birth to at least age twenty-two, investigators at the Fels Research Institute, Yellow Springs, Ohio, have found that full adult stature is reached and growth stops at a median age of 21.2 years in boys, 17.3 in girls. After age eighteen, very little further growth occurs: a median of slightly less than half an inch in boys, still less in girls.   (P-21)

Pinworm problems—including urinary infections

Common in children, pinworms usually produce itching around the rectal area. But a recent study by R. D. Simon of Walla Walla, Washington, indicates that the parasites may also be responsible for some urinary tract infections in girls. Of a group of girls, aged eighteen months to ten years, with urinary infections, 57 percent had pinworms. It appears possible for the worms to move from the rectal area through the short female urethra into the bladder, carrying along with them intestinal bacteria that may produce the urinary infection. Along with treatment for the bacterial infection, use of a standard anti-pinworm agent such as piperazine, pyrvinium pamoate, or thiabendazole, may be helpful in preventing repeated infection.   (P-22)

The hoarse and raspy voice

Some children develop hoarse, raspy voices because of nodules on their vocal cords. Most often, they are between the ages of five and ten years, are three times more likely to be boys than girls, and tend to be incessant talkers and shouters.

Reassuring facts come from a study of seventy-seven such children. With treatment by school speech therapists or other professionals, some children improved—but so did some who were getting no help at all.

Apparently, with or without help, the problem is self-limiting, over with at puberty, with nodules as well as hoarseness and raspiness disappearing at that time. All the children in the study who have reached puberty are free of the problem.   (P-23)

High blood pressure in childhood

High blood pressure, or hypertension, is one of the most common diseases of adults, the cause of as many as one-half of all deaths from heart and blood vessel diseases.

Because hypertension may begin early in life, more and more authorities now urge that blood pressure measurements should be— although they still are not—a regular and routine part of the physical examination of every child over the age of two, and even younger.

Although studies of hypertension in young children are relatively recent and have been carried out on only a small scale, they indicate that elevations of pressure may be present even in the very young.

In one study, carried out over a three-year period at the I. W. Killam Hospital for Children, Halifax, Nova Scotia, by Dr. John Crocker, eighty-five children were found to be hypertensive, nearly one-fourth of them under a year of age.

In about half of those under a year old and almost two-thirds of those somewhat older, a definite cause of the pressure elevation, most commonly a kidney problem, could be found. At all ages, control of markedly elevated pressure could be achieved readily with medical treatment. Surgery, when indicated for a definite cause, produced a high cure rate.

Curiously, some infants with hypertension of unknown cause, after six months of medical treatment, could stop taking medication and their pressures remained in the normal range.   (P-24)

Detecting and correcting other heart risk factors in children

Pediatricians and other physicians caring for children are being urged increasingly to make regular blood tests for cholesterol and to check on other risk factors as well as hypertension in their young patients.

In a study in which blood cholesterol was measured in more than two thousand healthy children, aged from two weeks to nineteen years, by Drs. Glenn M. Friedman and S. J. Goldberg of the University of Arizona College of Medicine, Tucson, 35 percent of youngsters over the age of nine were found to have levels that might be associated over a period of time with accumulation of fatty deposits in artery linings that could eventually lead to heart attacks and strokes. When a high cholesterol level is found in a child, the physicians report, parents can be advised of dietary changes that can keep the condition under control.   (P-25)

In another study of 4,829 children by Dr. R. M. Lauer and a team of pediatric cardiologists of University Hospitals, Iowa City, the mean cholesterol level at all ages proved to be 182, but 24 percent of the children had levels above 200, 9 percent above 220, 3 percent above 240, and 1 percent above 260.

Levels of blood fats (triglycerides) rose from a mean of 70 at age seven to 108 at age eighteen, but 15 percent of the children had levels of 140 or more.

In the Iowa study, no child under age nine had blood pressure greater than 140/90, considered top normal in adults. But after age fourteen, 8.9 percent had systolic pressure above 140, 12.2 percent had diastolic pressure above 90, and 4.4 percent had both pressures at or above these levels.

Obesity, another risk factor, was all too common. Between ages six and nine, 20 percent of children had weights 10 percent greater and 5 percent had weights 30 percent greater than the group as a whole. In the fourteen to eighteen age group, 25 percent had 10 percent and 8 percent had 30 percent greater weights than the group as a whole.

Thus a substantial number of children, the investigators warn, may show one or more risk factors that can and should be corrected. (P-26)

Avoiding dog bites

Each year, about half a million Americans are bitten by dogs and most victims are children. In as many as 90 percent of cases, the animals are not strange but rather are family pets or other known and previously friendly dogs. In almost every case, according to a study by Drs. A. B. Sokol and R. G. Houser of the Ohio State University Hospital, Columbus, a bitten child tries to pet the dog at an inopportune moment or startles, teases, or mistreats the animal.

Many bites could be avoided, the physicians report, if children are taught not only to stay away from strange dogs but also never to startle, tease, or mistreat a friendly one and to respect all dogs, especially when they are eating, sleeping, or eliminating.   (P-27)

Children and sports

Are school sports hazardous? To some extent, yes—but they are more beneficial than harmful. And, according to the American Medical Association's Committee on the Medical Aspects of Sports, because children tend to play rough and take chances anywhere—on gym floor, school athletic field, or in casual unsupervised play—their chances of being hurt are much less in supervised school sports.

Along with the increased safety of supervised school physical education and athletics, the committee reports, studies show that school sport participation provides learning-in-the-classroom benefits as well as improved physical fitness, with some contributions as well to social and emotional maturity.   (P-28)

What of prepubescent girls and boys competing against each other in sports, physical education, and recreational activities? There is no reason that they should not—except in heavy collision sports where, because of their lesser muscle mass per unit of body weight, girls risk serious injury, reports the American Academy of Pediatrics' Committee on the Pediatric Aspects of Physical Fitness, Recreation, and Sports.

Actually, however, the committee adds, the ultimate benefits are greater when girls—and women—have opportunities to engage in sports competition sponsored just for them. "Girls," the committee emphasizes, "can attain high levels of fitness through strenuous conditioning activities to improve their physical fitness, agility, strength, appearance, endurance and sense of psychic well-being," and, contrary to many misconceptions, such activities "have no unfavorable influence on menstruation, future pregnancy, and childbirth." (P-29)

CHAPTER 16

Respiratory Diseases

Asthma: the problem—and some new insights into causes

At least 1 percent of the American population—more than two million people—have some degree of asthma.

Air reaches the lungs through the bronchial tubes, which branch off from the windpipe, or trachea, and become smaller and smaller as they penetrate the depths of the lungs.

The tubes have muscular, elastic walls and soft, delicate linings containing many mucus-producing cells. In asthma, depending upon severity, there may be constriction of the tubes, swelling of the linings, and overproduction of mucus, and plugs of mucus may harden and block air passages.

An asthma attack may be so mild that a patient feels only a slight heaviness in breathing, or it may be so severe that the patient strains virtually every muscle of the upper body in attempts to get air in and out of the blocked bronchi. Breathing may be loud and wheezing, the lips blue from poor oxygenation of the blood, and the face may have the agonized look of someone suffocating. Most attacks are moderate, last a few hours, then clear. Between attacks, breathing is normal. After a severe attack, there may be chest muscle soreness from the labored breathing.

Asthma is considered to be, basically, an allergic disorder. But it has special characteristics that separate it from other allergic disorders. For example, asthma may cause permanent lung damage, whereas most allergies do not severely damage their target organs. Also, there have appeared to be stronger psychological factors in many cases of asthma than in other allergies, enough stronger so that asthma has been considered a psychosomatic as well as an allergic disorder. Moreover, asthma can be precipitated by factors other than allergic reactions and psychologic and emotional states.

The most common allergic causes of asthma

Recently, after thirty-seven years of experience with asthma in children, Dr. W. C. Deaner of the University of California School of Medicine, San Francisco, summed up his findings: that asthma is usually a preventable disease due to inhalants or foods or both; that emotional factors and bacterial infections are rarely the chief problems.

Among the most common inhalant causes in his experience are house dust, house dust mites, pollens, molds, and cat or dog dander. Skin tests are reliable in detecting these causes.

But unrecognized food allergy, Dr. Deaner has found, is the most frequent cause of unexplained asthma in children—for one thing, because skin tests are not completely reliable in detecting food allergens and, for another, because other symptoms that often accompany asthma, such as headaches, stomachaches, "growing pains," tiredness and fatigue, nervous tension, and pallor are seldom recognized as symptoms due to food allergy.

The most frequent troublemakers, accounting between them for half or more of food-caused asthma in children, Deaner has found, are milk (including cheese, ice cream, and sherbet that contain it) and chocolate (including cola drinks that contain a chocolate derivative).   (R-1)

Other reports recently indicate that shellfish, eggs, nuts, berries, and wheat are also among the most allergenic of foods. They indicate, too, that elimination diets—trials in which suspected foods are eliminated and gradually replaced until those that provoke asthma are determined—can be very helpful.   (R-2)

A cardinal principle of asthma management is environmental control of the patient's immediate living area—the bedroom. It should be as free of house dust and other airborne irritants as possible. It may be necessary in some cases to exclude household pets in order to eliminate dander—and indoor plants to eliminate mold spores.

It can also be important, recent reports emphasize, for an asthma patient to undergo a complete desensitization program involving injections of small doses of specific agents such as weed, grass, and tree pollens, and house dust to which he has been shown by skin tests to be allergic. The injections may build up greater tolerance.   (R-3)

Can emotional problems really cause asthma?

To find out, investigators at the National Asthma Center in Denver recently studied eighteen young asthmatic patients, boys between the ages of ten years six months and fourteen years ten months. They equipped the boys with little portable radio transmitters about cigarette pack size and had them go out and engage in usual play activities.

The transmitters picked up the youngsters' yelling, laughing, crying, and other "vocal behavior," and at a centrally located receiver the sounds were taped for study. And every twenty minutes, each boy's peak respiratory flow was measured by a technician (the lower the flow, the more imminent an attack of asthma).

Correlating the vocal behavior from the tapes with the respiratory flow measurements, the investigators found that seven boys had markedly lower peak flow rates after increased laughter, three after yelling. So vocal behavior could lead to decreased flow rate and presumably asthma.

Emotions picked up on the tapes could also be correlated with flow measurements. Five boys had markedly lower peak flow rates after anger or excitement. So in some cases drops in flow rates large enough to precipitate asthma could be related to emotions.

Then the investigators went a step farther, having clinical psychologists at the center independently evaluate the psychological adjustment of the eighteen boys, rating them from 1 (best adjustment) to 7 (worst adjustment).

It turned out that all the five boys whose flow rate drops correlated with emotion were of average or better adjustment while none of the four considered to have the worst adjustment showed any signs of emotionally induced drops in peak flow.

So it seems that a child whose asthma attacks are triggered by emotional stress doesn't by any means have to be considered psychologically maladjusted.   (R-4)

Other asthma causes

Asthma and sinus disease. At least in a few cases, asthma may be related to sinusitis and treatment for the sinus condition could help the asthma, according to one recent medical report.

The report tells of five patients studied by Drs. C. S. Phipatanakul and R. G. Slavin of the Saint Louis University School of Medicine. In these patients asthma apparently was produced by sinus disease.

In all five, the asthma disappeared after successful sinus treatment, with two of the patients responding to medical management and three requiring surgical drainage of the sinuses.   (R-5)

Asthma and hyperthyroidism. Hyperthyroidism—excessive activity of the thyroid gland—is well known, when it is severe enough, to produce a few or many such symptoms as profuse sweating, dislike of heat, palpitation, insomnia, nervousness, and excitability.

Now it seems that it can sometimes contribute to asthma and may be, when unrecognized, the reason patients with severe asthma attacks fail to respond to all usual anti-asthma measures.

A team of Providence, Rhode Island, physicians headed by Dr. G. A. Settipane have reported on a group of patients with intractable asthma who were found to have, at the same time, hyperthyroidism. Treatment for the gland disorder brought striking improvement in the asthma in every case.   (R-6)

Asthma and aspirin sensitivity. Although it is one of the most valuable and widely used drugs, aspirin does not agree with some people. In the general population, a small minority—about 0.2 percent or one in five hundred people—have an allergic sensitivity to aspirin and may develop symptoms such as nasal stuffiness or wheezing.

But sensitivity among asthmatics is much greater. In some recent studies, about 20 percent of severe adult asthmatics have been found intolerant of the drug. And in a very recent study of fifty severe asthmatic children, aged six to eighteen, Dr. Gary S. Rachelefsky and a University of California at Los Angeles School of Medicine team found that 28 percent were intolerant.

Of the fourteen aspirin-sensitive youngsters, nine had asthma attacks within thirty minutes after taking aspirin; one had attacks within an hour; the remaining four, after two hours. Eleven of the fourteen children continued to have breathing difficulty for the next twenty-four hours.

The study suggests that it might be well to eliminate use of aspirin in children with chronic asthma. Aspirin substitutes, such as acetaminophen, are readily available. (R-7)

A drug to prevent asthma attacks

Drugs in some variety have been used for controlling episodes of asthma. A newer drug, cromolyn sodium, developed and used in England since 1968 and introduced in the United States in 1973, is preventive.

Cromolyn has a unique action: when inhaled before exposure to allergenic materials, it inhibits allergic reaction. Although it has no effect after the onset of an acute attack of asthma, as a preventive agent it has partially or completely eliminated attacks in many children and adults.

An evaluation of long-term studies of cromolyn indicates that it has achieved an unusual record of safety, produces no intolerance, and on long-term treatment many patients have increased tolerance for exercise, reduced need for hospitalization, decreased interference with sleep, and lessened requirements for bronchodilators and corticosteroid drugs. (R-8)

The valuable ability of cromolyn, used before vigorous activity, to help make possible normal sporting and recreational pursuits, has been demonstrated in a study at the University of Western Australia. In more than three-fourths (77.2 percent) of asthma patients inhaling cromolyn fifteen minutes before exercise, the drug protected against exercise-induced asthma, and in those in whom asthma did occur as the result of exercise it was of shorter duration.

Importance of proper use. Cromolyn is unique not only in its action but also in its method of delivery. The drug in powder form is contained in a capsule. It is dispensed from a specially designed inhaler that punctures a capsule to release a fine mist of white powder that the patient inhales. This process permits the medication to reach the innermost portions of the lungs.

Improper use, a late medical report indicates, may be to blame in many cases in which cromolyn has failed to benefit patients. The report emphasizes several critical points:

1. Some chronic asthma patients have large amounts of mucus and may not be able to inhale adequate amounts of the powder into the lower bronchi. They should use a bronchodilating drug, delivered by a nebulizer, ideally for about a week even before beginning cromolyn and then about one-half hour before inhaling the powder. They should also be encouraged to cough before using cromolyn.

2. Patients should hold their breath as long as possible after inhalation to permit the powder to settle on the mucous membrane.

3. Before exhaling, patients should remove the inhaler from the mouth in order to prevent clumping of the powder.

4. Frequent washing with warm water of the propeller in the device, including the inside of the shaft, is advisable.

The report urges that the physician, nurse, or technician should make certain not only at the beginning but thereafter as well that a patient is using the device properly by having him repeatedly demonstrate how he uses it.   (R-9)

Symptomatic treatments for asthma

Several classes of drugs can be used in the management of asthma symptoms.

Bronchodilators are among the most widely used. They relax the bronchial muscles.

One of the many bronchodilators is theophylline which, when taken every six hours in carefully prescribed individualized dosages, is reported to be effective in many children with chronic asthma.

Other useful bronchodilators include epinephrine, isoproterenol, and ephedrine, which may be taken by mouth, by aerosol spray, or by injection. Some recently introduced drugs in the same class—metaproterenol sulfate and terbutaline sulfate—which can be administered by aerosol or injection—have been reported to be longer-acting and in some cases more effective.

Corticosteroid drugs may be used for patients who do not do well enough with bronchodilators, environmental control, and perhaps even with hyposensitization (anti-allergy injection treatment).

In the experience of more and more asthma specialists, the most satisfactory way to use corticosteroids is on an alternate-day basis. With an entire dose taken one morning and no more until another entire dose is taken forty-eight hours later, undesirable side effects are greatly reduced. Many experts believe that only the shorter-acting corticosteroids—prednisone, prednisolone, and methyl-prednisolone—should be used because they have the least tendency to suppress the normal functioning of the adrenal glands. In children, too, alternate day therapy is much less likely to interfere with growth.

(R-10)

Asthma control during pregnancy

For some women with severe asthma, corticosteroids may be the only means of control. But can the drugs be used safely during pregnancy?

A study to help answer that question was carried out by teams of Northwestern University, Chicago, and University of Washington, Seattle, physicians. They followed fifty-five asthmatic mothers requiring corticosteroid treatment through seventy pregnancies.

There were seventy-one live births (including two sets of twins) and only one miscarriage. There were no maternal deaths, no deaths of babies after birth, no increased incidence of toxemia or uterine hemorrhage in the mothers or congenital deformities in the infants.

When required for severe asthma, corticosteroids do not appear to noticeably increase risk for either mothers or children and should not be contraindicated during pregnancy, the physicians report.   (R-11)

Some special notes on asthmatic children and exercise

Provided it is the right kind, exercise, including active sports, often can be doubly helpful for asthmatic children. It may actually help with symptoms and, in addition, can be important in preventing feelings of isolation and inferiority that children may develop when they are left out of sports and many normal activities.

Guidelines—useful for physicians and parents—come from a recent study by the Committee on Rehabilitation Therapy of the American Academy of Allergy.

It is important that the exercise and sports be "proper," the study emphasizes.

Brief exercise—for one to two minutes—often decreases airway obstruction, and the more severe the obstruction before exercise, the greater the improvement afterward.

But more prolonged exercise—four minutes or longer—often has the opposite effect, causing constriction of breathing passages.

Therefore, suggests the committee, an asthmatic child should be encouraged to participate in such sports as baseball and sprint running that involve brief, vigorous activity but not in others such as basketball and long-distance running that require prolonged exertion.

Another recent study indicates that a combination of three drugs can allow many asthmatic youngsters to engage more fully in recreational and sports activities without suffering from attacks brought on by vigorous activity.

In a controlled study at the University of Washington, Seattle, physicians gave the drugs—ephedrine, theophylline, and hydroxyzine hydrochloride (a tranquilizing agent with some antihistamine and antispasmodic properties)—to children who wheezed after strenuous exercise. The drugs were tried separately and in combinations. Results were also compared with those after use of inert medication (placebo).

Both theophylline and ephedrine proved to be superior to placebo when given alone, even more effective in combination, and still more effective when hydroxyzine was added to the combination.   (R-12)

Hypnotherapy for asthma?

Can hypnotherapy be at all helpful to asthmatics?

A report reaching here from Australia suggests that it can be to a greater or lesser extent in some cases.

Hypnotherapy was tried in 121 asthmatic patients, all requiring regular treatment. Twenty-five (21 percent), most of them under age twenty, became free of asthma and required no drug treatment. Forty others (33 percent) showed a 50 percent or greater decrease in the frequency and severity of attacks and in drug requirements. Twenty-seven (22 percent) had what was classified as a poor response, with less than 50 percent improvement, and the remaining 29 (24 percent) showed no change.   (R-13)

The common cold: new insights into how you get it

"Coughs and sneezes spread diseases," according to an old saying. They may be involved in some, but new evidence indicates that if you recoil from every common cold sufferer you may well be recoiling without good cause; that catching a cold is more difficult than it was thought; and that colds are more likely to be spread by fingers or hands, and your best chance for avoiding a cold may be to be a "touch-me-not."

The Wisconsin couple surprise. To the surprise of the investigators at the University of Wisconsin, a study there with twenty-four married couples suggests that the prevailing idea that the common cold spreads like wildfire from person to person may be as much of a myth as the old belief that wet feet and a chill make for colds.

The twenty-four couples, most of them students at the university, volunteered to risk a cold in the interest of science. One person in each couple was infected by instilling nose drops containing a cold virus.

Duly the infected persons came down with colds. But only a minority of them—roughly 38 percent—transmitted their colds to their spouses. In the cases of transmission, the original cold was moderate or severe rather than mild in symptoms and the transmission took a lot of togetherness; where the spouses became infected, the couples spent many hours together, more than seventeen a day.

The study was undertaken because of the impression from citywide surveys, including one in Madison, Wisconsin, that person-to-person spread of virus was unpredictable even with respiratory virus infections widespread in a whole community. And the study confirmed the impression.   (R-14)

Another study provides an added insight.

The cold touch. Evidence that colds are far more likely to be transmitted by fingers or hands—by direct skin-to-skin contact or even by touching cold-virus-contaminated surfaces—than by sneeze or cough comes from a study by University of Virginia School of Medicine, Charlottesville, researchers.

The study established that in only two of twenty-five people with naturally acquired colds was any virus expelled in a cough or sneeze. On the other hand, in 40 percent of individuals with colds, the viruses were shed onto their hands.

Moreover, it turned out that the viruses on the hands could be transmitted to almost anything touched. The researchers were able to recover active viruses for up to three hours after they were deposited on wood, stainless steel and Formica surfaces, and from such synthetic fabrics as Dacron and nylon. The viruses seemed to be less long-lasting on porous fabrics such as cotton cloth and facial tissue.

Drying in itself had little effect on the viability of the virus. Virus dried on plastic was transferred to fingers touching the contaminated area in fifteen out of sixteen trials, and virus dried on the skin was transferred to fingers in three out of five trials. Four out of eleven people got colds after touching their nasal mucosa with fingers that had been contaminated by rubbing a dried drop of virus.

Going further to demonstrate that such transmission could occur under practical circumstances, the Virginia investigators checked into the amount of nose-picking and eye-rubbing in 124 adults—medical students and doctors attending a lecture, another group attending Sunday School—none of whom knew they were being observed.

Per hour of observation, one of every three subjects picked his nose and one of every 2.7 rubbed his eyes. For what it might be worth, the investigators found out that the physicians and medical students picked their noses nine times more often than did the Sunday School group but both groups rubbed their eyes with equal frequency.

The study thus suggests that it should be possible to avoid the spread of many colds—especially when one appears in a family—by avoidance of eye-rubbing and nose-picking, and that hand-washing may be more important than covering up coughs and sneezes. (R-15)

Common colds and other respiratory illnesses: Who gets them? When?

The better educated you are, the more colds likely; and the less well off you are, the more colds, too.

These are two of a series of findings emerging from a study by University of Michigan scientists of 4,905 Tecumseh, Michigan, residents who, over a six-year period, had 14,600 episodes of respiratory illness.

An explanation for the higher incidence of colds and other respiratory troubles among the poor could easily be crowded living that increases the likelihood of transmission of infectious diseases. But why higher incidence among the better educated? Possibly, suggest the investigators, the better educated have a tendency to recognize minor symptoms and consider that they indicate disease.

Other study findings:

As age increases, the annual illness rate decreases, except during the years twenty through twenty-nine, when it increases. After twenty-nine, the decline resumes.

Highest mean rate of illnesses—6.1 a year—occurs among infants under one year of age. And at less than a year of age and also from one year to two years, boys have more episodes of illness than do girls, but at age three and later girls get sick more often.

More illnesses begin on Monday than on any other days. That is particularly true for school-age children. And the illnesses can be real enough, occurring on Monday because infection in school would be transmitted during the first days of the school week and, following a period of incubation, the infection symptoms would pop up over the weekend.   (R-16)

Vitamin C for colds: Does it do any good? How much? Latest studies

Ever since 1970, when Nobel Laureate Linus Pauling published his book *Vitamin C and the Common Cold,* advocating large doses of the vitamin to prevent and treat colds, the debate over its merits has raged.

Almost every new study—and there have been many—has tended to fan rather than resolve the controversy.

In one of the latest, reported to a Stanford University Symposium on Vitamin C, 641 Navajo boarding-school students were divided into two groups by Drs. J. L. Coulehan, K. S. Reisinger, and K. D. Rogers of Fort Defiance Hospital in Arizona. Some children received a high intake of vitamin C—1 or 2 grams (1,000 to 2,000 milligrams)—per day over a period of time while others, for comparison, received inert medication (placebo).

Overall, in those receiving it, the vitamin led to a 30 percent reduction in days of sickness from respiratory illness. There were 34 percent fewer days of sickness in children aged ten to fifteen, and 28 percent fewer in children aged six to ten.

Although it reduced total sick days from colds, the vitamin did not cut the incidence of colds.

An extra dividend indicated by the study: total days of sickness from *nonrespiratory* problems among younger children fell by 30 percent with use of vitamin C.   (R-17)

Another study, reported a few months later, was carried out by University of Toronto investigators to determine whether vitamin C in relatively low doses had any influence on the burden of winter illness.

Participating in the study were 622 volunteers, all in general good health but usually afflicted with at least one cold each winter. Some received vitamin C in a dose of just 500 milligrams once a week, and 1,500 milligrams on the first day and 1,000 milligrams on the next four days of any illness. Others received inert pills for comparison.

The volunteers on the vitamin had less severe illness, with about 25 percent fewer days spent indoors because of illness.

The results, suggest the investigators, support the idea that vitamin C can reduce the drag of winter illness but the intake apparently doesn't have to be as high as often claimed.   (R-18)

The latest from Dr. Pauling on vitamin C and the cold

Altogether, since the publication of Pauling's book in 1970, thirteen controlled trials have been carried out in which some subjects received vitamin C (100 milligrams or more per day) and others received a placebo.

Recently, Pauling reviewed the studies. Seven in his opinion were good studies, carefully set up from the scientific standpoint; the other six were flawed.

The seven good studies—including the two already mentioned and others carried out in Canada, Scotland, and Switzerland—show decreases in the amount of illness ranging from 25 percent to 68 percent, and an average reduction in illness by vitamin C of 44 percent. The six other studies, considered less reliable by Pauling, gave an average protection of 19 percent.

"There is accordingly," writes Dr. Pauling, "overwhelming evidence that the regular ingestion of supplementary vitamin C provides some protection against the common cold, decreasing the amount of illness by nearly half.

"I believe, however, that a far greater amount of protection can be obtained by adjusting the intake of vitamin C to the circumstances. I think that every person needs at least 200 milligrams per day for really good health, and that the optimum daily dose for most people is larger. A gram a day or more.

"These regular doses will block most colds, but not all. If you feel tired or listless or are under some strain, take one or two grams more, and continue every hour until you feel better. It is especially important to begin this high hourly intake at the very first sign of a cold—the first sneeze, shiver, or drop of nasal secretion. Usually your body can then stop the cold—which no cold medicine can do. Even if the cold is not stopped, the high intake of vitamin C (totalling 10 to 30 grams in a day) will ameliorate it so greatly that you will have much less suffering than with your usual colds. Also, you will be in much less danger of contracting a secondary bacterial infection and developing mastoiditis, meningitis, or other serious disease.

"If you begin to catch a cold and treat it by an increased intake of vitamin C so that you feel better, do not then drive yourself to extra exertion, or the cold may succeed in overcoming your defenses. Instead, live an easy life for a day or two, while you continue your high intake of the vitamin."

Dr. Pauling has this to say about the *kind* of vitamin C to use: "The best vitamin C to use is the cheapest. Pure crystalline powder vitamin C can be purchased retail for as little as $9.85 per kilogram (1,000 grams), and 1-gram tablets for $22 per kilogram. There is no need to buy rose-hip or acerola vitamin C at $40 or more per kilogram. A level teaspoon of the vitamin in crystalline powder form is 4.4 grams. Use a set of measuring spoons for precision in taking the quantity you desire."   (R-19)

Croup: a simple first aid measure

An acute attack of spasmodic croup in a child can be frightening to both parents and child. Typically, it occurs at night and onset is sudden, with hoarse, "croupy" voice or cough and breathing difficulty. It most often affects two- to four-year-olds after a mild upper respiratory infection with slight temperature elevation.

A simple home measure can bring quick initial relief until the child can be seen by a physician, advises Dr. Adam G. N. Moore of Squantum, Massachusetts.

He suggests that a parent turn on the cold shower in the bathroom and then sit down in the room with the child held comfortably in sitting position on the lap. "The cold mist and the upright posture both help immensely and can be followed up by either an office visit or a house call."   (R-20)

New help for virus croup

Also known as acute laryngotracheobronchitis, so-called virus croup often enough is caused by virus infection but may also be by strep, staph, and other bacteria. Occurring most often in late winter or early spring, it may appear at any age but most often affects infants and children. It may develop during the course of what has seemed to be a cold or may strike the apparently well.

Mucous membranes of the larynx, trachea, and bronchi are inflamed. Edema, or water-logging of tissues, is severe and this, along with copious, sticky mucus that is constantly secreted, can threaten to block breathing passages.

Each year, about forty-seven thousand children with severe laryngotracheobronchitis require hospitalization. In about fifteen hundred, standard treatment—including use of a mist-filled oxygen tent, antibiotics, and other medication—is not enough and emergency tracheotomies, or throat incisions, are needed to prevent suffocation.

Tracheotomies, however, may often be avoidable, one study indicates, with a new treatment: inhalation of a drug, vaporized racemic epinephrine, in a respirator.

At Primary Children's Hospital, Salt Lake City, the treatment has been found to work within fifteen minutes, clearing tracheal blockage and ending the threat of suffocation.

According to a report from the hospital, the treatment has reduced tracheotomies to zero, no fatalities have occurred in more than three hundred croup cases, and almost one-third of youngsters receiving the treatment in the hospital emergency room could be sent home without being hospitalized.   (R-21)

How to breath downtown air

In large amounts, of course, carbon monoxide can be lethal—and fast. But even in small amounts, it is a hazard to health, receiving increasing recognition in particular as a possibly hazardous factor for the heart.

Because busy downtown streets have been found to have very high concentrations of carbon monoxide from motor vehicle exhausts, University of Toronto investigators have studied how exposure to the invisible, odorless gas can be minimized when you go into downtown areas to work or shop.

Their suggestions: As a pedestrian, you will usually do best to choose the windward side of the street—the side from which the wind is blowing—and to walk as far from the curb as you can. If a still air zone is created by a tall building or construction walkway, cross to the opposite side of the street if possible.

If you ride a bicycle, you're likely to be at higher risk because of faster, deeper breathing from the effort of riding and especially if you ride behind exhaust pipes of cars, trucks, and buses. By all means, when possible, choose less congested streets. And at traffic lights, either move ahead of the exhaust pipe of the first vehicle or hold well back of the last vehicle until the lights change.   (R-22)

CHAPTER 17

Skin, Hair, and Nails

Acne: New approaches to combatting it

Acne, a persistent, sometimes scarring and disfiguring disease, most often attacks young people but is hardly limited to them.

One important new development in treatment has been the finding that a form of vitamin A—vitamin A acid cream (Retin-A)—has the effect of repressing formation of blackheads and unseating existing ones. It does this by promoting peeling and shedding of affected outer skin layers, thus unplugging impacted pores.

The preparation alone often is sufficient when acne is mild or blackheads are the main problem.

But it has to be used properly, and too often physicians do not do a thorough job of explaining to patients exactly how to use it, reports Dr. Albert M. Kligman, a dermatologist of the University of Pennsylvania School of Medicine, Philadelphia, who did much of the research with the vitamin and is noted for other innovative research.

There are several possible problem areas in using the drug:

1. Vitamin A acid causes some redness and peeling. Excessive use will bring swelling and intense redness. The patient needs careful instruction in the daily amount of application that will induce mild redness and peeling but will not be an overdose.

2. Skin that is peeling from vitamin A acid is particularly quick to sunburn, and patients should be advised about this and cautioned to stay out of the sun or use a sunscreen preparation.

3. The color of the skin may lighten somewhat after long use of the drug. This is seldom important and is not permanent but the patient should be advised that it might happen.   (S-1)

When acne is severe and pustules numerous, a combination of vitamin A acid applied to the skin and an antibiotic, demeclocycline hydrochloride, taken internally often produces excellent results.

The two measures complement each other's effectiveness through a double attack on the processes that contribute to acne. As vitamin A acid clears the pores, the antibiotic relieves the inflammation and redness.

Results in a study with a large group of adolescents using the combination indicate that once the acne is under control with the combination, the antibiotic dosage can be reduced and finally stopped while vitamin A acid can be used indefinitely until the skin clearance is permanent.   (S-2)

Still other work by the University of Pennsylvania investigators is promising for the future.

Vitamin A acid has been used, in studies in Philadelphia, along with a special lotion form of an antibiotic, erythromycin.

The inflammation in severe acne is incited by bacteria. Destroying the bacteria can reduce the inflammation. But the problem has been to get an antibiotic drug to the bugs. Antibiotics taken by mouth get there through the bloodstream. Theoretically, an antibiotic applied directly to the skin could get there faster.

But until now topical antibiotics for acne have not worked well. Erythromycin does. At least half the acne in 80 percent of patients cleared over an eight-week period.

The antibiotic in its lotion form penetrates the skin more effectively than other antibiotics such as tetracycline and chloramphenicol.

But the problem at the moment is that erythromycin in topical form is not commercially available. In that form, it is unstable. For the

Philadelphia studies, new batches had to be specially prepared every two weeks.

How soon it will be commercially available is not known. The University of Pennsylvania investigators believe, however, that pharmaceutical companies have the ability to develop a stable form useful for the skin.   (S-3)

Use of liquid nitrogen is another newer approach reported to show promise—not for less severe forms of acne with blackheads and pimples but for severe pustular acne.

In a study by Dr. D. K. Goette of Walter Reed Army Medical Center, Washington, D.C., liquid nitrogen was applied once a week to one side of the face of twenty-five patients and results were compared with conventional topical applications of various kinds applied to the other side.

Liquid nitrogen had no advantage in milder acne with pimples and blackheads. But in eight of eleven patients with pustular acne, it was notably effective, with pustules clearing within two to three days, leaving only some redness for another four to five days.   (S-4)

Acne and food: any real connection?

It has long been assumed by many physicians as well as by acne victims and their families that certain foods can trigger or exacerbate acne. The prime suspected culprits: chocolate, nuts, cola, milk, cheese, butter, fried foods, iodized salt.

Rather than take this for granted, Dr. Philip C. Anderson of the University of Missouri-Columbia School of Medicine carried out an investigation, selecting acne victims who were convinced that their skin condition worsened substantially, and usually within thirty-six hours, after eating some particular food.

Every day for a week, at a clinic, each patient was fed large amounts of the food supposed in each case to be bad. Both before and after the week-long study, each patient's facial appearance was mapped in detail: acne lesions were counted, located and graded according to size, depth, and severity.

To the considerable surprise not only of the patients but also of medical students helping in the study, the suspected foods led to no major flares of acne.

According to Anderson, it is quite likely that physical

disturbances—tension, fatigue, loss of sleep, indigestion—can play some part in acne, but the study indicates that the suspected foods contribute little if at all.

Of some concern to Anderson: the possibility that myths about foods and acne may lead some victims to use bizarre, potentially harmful diets. "Our university nutritionist," he has reported, "has shown me that common goiter is increasing among teen-agers, some of whom were using noniodized salt to prevent acne."   (S-5)

Acne, other skin problems, and oral contraceptives

Women with severe acne may benefit from birth control pills because the estrogen component of the pills tends to reduce oil secretions that have a "fueling" effect on acne, investigators have found. Commonly, several months are required before any beneficial effects may become apparent, and in the first two months there may even be a temporary increase in acne, but thereafter continued use may produce improvement.   (S-6)

But investigators have also noted differences between various oral contraceptive preparations and their effects on acne. Some are estrogen-dominant, but others are progestogen-dominant, and while the former may help improve acne, the latter may exacerbate it.

At the University of Oklahoma, Dr. V. P. Barranco has reported on a group of women whose acne had worsened on progestogen-dominant oral contraceptives. When they were switched to estrogen-dominant pills, more than 90 percent showed slight improvement in two months and marked improvement in four months.   (S-7)

At the Western Gynecological and Obstetrical Clinic, Salt Lake City, Utah, Dr. H. G. McQuarrie also has found that choice of a pill with a suitable combination of the hormones estrogen and progestogen can minimize or avoid acne or other skin effects.

For women who have acne or develop it while on an oral contraceptive, he advises use of a contraceptive that is more estrogenic rather than a progestationally dominant one such as norethindrone, norgestrel, or norethindrone acetate.

A more estrogenic contraceptive is also useful when the problem is abnormal hairiness (hypertrichosis).

On the other hand, for darkening of skin pigmentation, a frequent cosmetic nuisance that may stem from oral contraceptives, a pill very low in, or entirely free of, estrogen may help.   (S-8)

Stirring up skin problems with steroid creams

Steroids—cortisonelike drugs—in cream form, when expertly used, can be valuable in some skin problems such as intertrigo and disabling contact dermatitis.

But they can be worse than useless, adding to original trouble or producing new trouble, when applied for trivial disorders.

A report by University of Pennsylvania physicians indicates that common misusers are women who apply the preparations for such problems as acne, aging changes, or "bad complexion."

To begin with, the original problem may improve somewhat—only for the improvement to be followed by complications. Acne is one. A rosacea-like condition, with bright red cheeks, is another. A third: perioral dermatitis—appearance around the mouth of small papules on a red, sometimes scaling, background.

To combat these complications, steroid use must be eliminated, and it may be necessary as well that an antibiotic, tetracycline, be taken by mouth.   (S-9)

Athlete's foot: new understanding, better treatment

Also known as tinea pedis, and ringworm of the foot, athlete's foot can be a stubbornly resistant nuisance affliction. At its height, with soggy, malodorous, whitish, itching between-the-toes lesions, it can be distracting.

Supposedly, the whole problem lies with a fungus, a microscopic plant growth, that thrives in locker rooms, public showers, and swimming pool walkways—and on the dead cells of the skin between the toes.

But that, it turns out from recent research, is a half-truth. Although athlete's foot starts out as a fungal infection, it then produces no symptoms, only some dry scaling.

When it becomes really troublesome—with odor, itching, and other annoying symptoms—the fungi are no longer active and may not even be present. Bacteria are the culprits.

Even some years ago, investigators at both Johns Hopkins University and the University of Pennsylvania discovered that in 75 percent of typical, advanced, symptomatic cases they could not recover any fungi at all.

Now, very recently, at the University of Pennsylvania, researchers have put together a picture of what happens:

First comes fungus infection with the fungi propagating between the toes, leading to some scaling of skin there. Then, at some point, excessive moisture is introduced—because of exercise, hot weather, tight shoes, or even emotionally induced excessive sweating.

The moisture is ideal for bacteria, including some previously harmless types normally residing in relatively small numbers between the toes. The bacteria multiply thanks to the moisture and drive out the fungi. And the bacteria produce the acute symptoms.

This being the case, the investigators decided, what was needed was some preparation that could assure drying. If it could also have a broad antibacterial action, that would be all to the good.

A search for a possibly suitable preparation finally narrowed to a series of aluminum compounds—aluminum chloride, aluminum chlorohydroxide, aluminum sulfate, and a few others—some of them previously used as antiperspirants.

With the help of prisoner volunteers in Philadelphia, all suffering from severe athlete's foot, the compounds in various concentrations were tried.

The most effective proved to be a solution of 30 percent aluminum chloride ($AlCl_36H_2O$), which any druggist can prepare at a cost of about two to three dollars for four ounces.

In the Philadelphia study, the solution, applied twice a day with a cotton-tipped applicator, relieved itching and ended malodor within forty-eight to seventy-two hours, and led to marked abatement of all symptoms within a week.

Only rarely does the preparation produce irritation. In cases where this has occurred, a fissure—a narrow, deep slit—has been present, allowing the solution to penetrate deeply, below the scaling and horny skin, to living skin. So in uncommon cases where fissures are present, the solution should not be used.

Usually, the solution can be used until complete clearance has occurred. Thereafter, it may be necessary to use it only once a day in especially hot, humid weather.   (S-10)

Relief for dry skin foot conditions

Persistent dry skin conditions of the feet from varied causes including fungal infections and ichthyosis (with its dryness, roughness, and scaliness resulting from failure of normal shedding of the keratin produced by skin cells) often can be helped by urea, a compound that increases water uptake by the stratum corneum portion of the skin and also has a useful, mild peeling action on the horny skin layer.

In one study, by Dr. Donald P. Nash, a San Francisco podiatrist, every one of seventy-five patients benefited from use of a urea preparation (Carmol Cream) with relief of itching, fissuring of heels, cracking, and other symptoms. The preparation also promoted healing.

(S-11)

Honey and the skin

Can natural honey when applied under a dry dressing help bring about healing of bedsores and burns? Better, reports one English physician, Dr. Robert Blomfield of Chelsea, than any other local application he has ever used. It is also, he finds, an inexpensive and valuable cleansing and healing agent for cuts, abrasions, and other surface wounds—one, he adds, that even has a delicious taste. (S-12)

A gum for bedsores

Because bedsores, or decubitus ulcers, often are notably difficult to eliminate, many treatments have been tried. A new, reportedly quite effective one, developed by an innovative nurse at the Louisville, Kentucky, Veterans Administration Hospital, makes use of karaya vegetable gum, once used as a remedy for other problems and still to be found on hospital stockroom shelves.

After applying antiseptic to the ulcer and surrounding skin, she applies a karaya gum ring to the skin, molding it to fit around the edge of the ulcer, sprinkles karaya powder on the sore, applies a polyurethane foam pad that covers the sore and the gum ring to avoid pressure on the ulcer, then covers the whole area with plastic kitchen wrap. She reports that the average time for healing is as little as a week for superficial ulcers.   (S-13)

Zinc for chronic leg sores

The metal zinc is one of a class of substances—trace elements— present in the body in the tiniest amounts. Recent studies have demonstrated that zinc is vital for many purposes. One of them is wound healing. Among the first studies were those done with otherwise-healthy young airmen recovering from surgery. All received the same treatment but half also received zinc in the form of zinc sulfate to take by mouth. In the zinc-treated, healing time was halved.

More recently, a Swedish study at Lund Hospital, Stockholm, indicates that zinc sulfate taken orally often may improve the healing of chronic venous leg sores.

Investigators there found low levels of zinc in the blood of fourteen patients with the sores. Seven then were given zinc sulfate and, for comparison, seven others received inert tablets. In those getting the zinc, zinc blood levels rose to normal in six weeks and remained normal; in the others, the levels remained low. During eighteen weeks of treatment, the sores healed in five of the seven zinc-treated patients, in only one of the patients receiving inert tablets.   (S-14)

Zinc for a grave baby rash

A long-mysterious disorder that manifests itself in some babies at weaning can be life-threatening. It may, at first, seem to be much like diaper rash, but the rash thickens and spreads from buttocks to leg, face, and elsewhere. Hair loss, diarrhea, and weight loss also develop.

After recently discovering gross zinc deficiency in such infants, suggesting that the explanation for the disorder (called acrodermatitis enteropathica) could be an inherited zinc deficiency, Dr. Edmund J. Moynahan at Guy's Hospital, London, tried giving about 35 milligrams of zinc sulfate a day to a group of babies with the condition. "All," he has reported, "are now completely symptom-free and are thriving on the zinc supplement."   (S-15)

Zinc and the fingernails

Not uncommonly, children and teen-agers and some adults as well have numerous queer white spots in the fingernails. They sometimes occur in toenails as well.

In a recent report, investigators at the Brain Bio Center, Princeton, New Jersey, suggest that the spots may be mainly the result of a zinc-deficient diet.

They also note that, using a zinc supplement along with vitamin B_6, they have been able to clear smaller white spots and prevent further spot formation. Large spots, however, have to grow out with the nails over a period of five to six months.   (S-16)

Hair transplantation

More than one million transplants of hair have been made since the technique was first devised twenty years ago by Dr. Norman Orentreich of New York City.

The success rate for survival of transplanted hair, when the procedure is carried out by a trained surgeon, now approaches 100 percent. There have been poor results, however, in the past—with a national average for graft survival of only about 40 percent as little as five years ago—traceable largely to doctors who undertook to do the seemingly simple procedure without learning very much about it.

A plug of hair is punched out from an area where hair is growing well and transferred to a bald area. One plug commonly contains eight or nine hairs but may contain as many as fifteen if the hair is fine. Commonly, too, the maximum number of plugs per square inch is twenty to twenty-five. From ten to fifty plugs may be grafted in a session.

Surgeons may differ somewhat in technique. Many punch out the plugs by hand. Some use a special power-driven cutter operated at slow speeds. This may allow more plugs—as many as fifty to seventy—to be grafted in one session.

Some surgeons prefer not to do transplantation in young men still losing their hair but would rather wait until hair loss is completed and the patients are as bald as they ever would be without transplants. Others, however, favor early hairline restoration in young adults. The transplants may be begun as soon as thinning is noticeable if the hair loss is only in the crown area. If the hairline is receding or if both hairline and crown are affected, reconstruction of the frontal hairline first is favored by some surgeons. They may begin transplants when the hairline has receded to a point where the man feels he would be satisfied if it were possible to prevent further recession. The hairline can be strengthened at this point and grafts can be implanted to replace hair loss as it continues, both in back of the reconstructed hairline and in the crown.   (S-17)

For the completely bald

A sizeable number of men are completely, or almost completely, bald so that they have no scalp hair to be used for grafting.

Recently, the original developer of the transplant technique, Dr. Norman Orentreich of the Orentreich Medical Group in New York City, has been experimenting with homografts—hair plugs taken from others for implantation in the bald.

As with grafts of donated tissues and organs elsewhere in the body, there is an immunosuppression or rejection problem. After trying other approaches to preventing rejection, Orentreich has resorted to injection of corticosteroids (cortisonelike drugs) directly into the site of a transplant. The injections have to be continued once a month to keep the grafts going. Some patients who have volunteered for trials of the technique have retained their donated hair thus far for as long as three years.   (S-18)

Other uses for hair transplants

First used for common male baldness, hair transplants more recently have been proving helpful for other types of hair loss—from scars, burns, accidents, operations, radiation, infections, and systemic diseases.

In addition to scalp hair loss, they have been used to remedy eyebrow loss, reports Dr. Robert Auerbach of New York University School of Medicine, with continuing good results, suggesting that the grafts will continue to function effectively for a lifetime.   (S-19)

Bald spots in women: traction alopecia

Traction alopecia—hair loss traceable to hard pulling on the hair—occurs in some women who use certain types of hairdos.

The problem is a preventable one, and, when recognized in time for what it is, a remediable one, report Drs. Francis S. Renna and Irwin M. Freedberg of Harvard Medical School, Boston.

Actually, traction alopecia was first reported among Greenland women using a particular type of coiffure. Traditional Japanese hairdos also have been blamed for bald areas. European physicians also have noted that baldness begins to develop along the frontal hairline in women who pull their hair back into a tight bun.

Hard pulling on hair shafts, as with tight bobby pins, also can lead to hair loss and bald spots, the Harvard physicians report. One of their patients, a nurse, developed what seemed at first to be two mysterious small bald spots. It turned out that those were the two points where she used bobby pins to hold her nurse's cap on her head. When she varied placement of the pins, instead of using them in the same locations every day, the hair gradually reappeared.

If traction or pull is eliminated as soon as baldness appears, the Boston physicians find, the hair usually grows back, but if the traction is continued, the hair loss may become permanent.   (S-20)

Surgery for uncontrollable underarm perspiration

Excessive underarm sweating, resistant to all the usual measures, can be a psychologically as well as aesthetically disturbing condition.

A recent report from Danish surgeons published here in the *Journal of the American Medical Association* offers new hope for victims.

It breaks down the results of a relatively simple new operation that removes underarm sweat glands—relatively simple because up to 80 percent of the glands are concentrated in a small area.

Mostly in the last two years, more than 250 people have had the operation, men and women mainly in the twenty- to forty-year age group and troubled with excessive perspiration since early youth.

Of more than one hundred patients who have been followed up and checked, 64 percent are completely satisfied with results; 29 percent a little less so, but pleased; 7 percent are dissatisfied.   (S-21)

New medical treatment for previously uncontrollable underarm perspiration

Within months after the report on surgery (above) appeared, another detailing a new medical approach to the problem appeared, also in the *Journal of the American Medical Association.*

At the Hospital of the University of Pennsylvania, Philadelphia, Drs. Walter B. Shelley and Harry J. Hurley, Jr., have been able to achieve sustained underarm dryness with a topical preparation—20 percent aluminum chloride hexahydrate in anhydrous ethyl alcohol (200 proof).

It has proved regularly effective, they report, in patients following their instructions: to apply the preparation at bedtime to the dried, unwashed underarm area; cover the area with a plastic sheeting such as Saran Wrap kept snug against the skin with a dress-shield garment or well-fitted body sheet; and, in the morning, remove the plastic and wash the area.

Thereafter, they find, a once-a-week application keeps the area dry indefinitely.   (S-22)

Drying the sweaty palm

Excessive sweating of the palm can also be a disturbing problem. An effective method of treatment has been reported by Dr. H. H. Gordon of the Southern California Permanente Medical Group, Fontana, California.

A 10 percent aqueous glutaraldehyde solution, not alkalinized, he found, is a rapidly effective antiperspirant for the palms. Its chief disadvantage: staining.

After experience with many patients, however, he has found that a 5 percent starting strength of the solution, rather than 10 percent, used three times a week, minimizes the staining. Thereafter, a maintenance strength of 2½ percent or less, used as necessary, is effective.

Although there is a possibility of an allergic reaction to glutaraldehyde, Gordon reports, no patient treated thus far has developed it.   (S-23)

Itching

Itching can stem from an extremely wide range of problems. Inordinate itching can come from flea bites, fungus and yeast infections, ringworm, the hives of allergy, and eczema. A few serious disorders such as obstructive jaundice, diabetes, kidney disorder, and internal cancer may be associated with itching. Itching also occurs with some forms of anemia.

Among numerous external causes of itching are tight or irritating clothing, reactions to insecticides, paint or varnish, dusts, fiber glass, dyes, and even the overlong and overhot baths sometimes used by arthritics.

Scratching only seems to relieve the discomfort. Actually, scratching, unfortunately, lowers the itch threshold and commonly brings on a cycle of itching, scratching, more itching, more scratching. Some people pinch the skin next to the itching site to get relief. Some apply extreme cold which stops the itching temporarily but seems to be followed by more intense itching.

When itching is complicated, experts report, medical help is needed and referral to a dermatologist, or skin specialist, may be advisable.

When, however, the itching problem is not too complicated, suggests one medical journal editorial, this recommendation may work: "If the skin is dry, moisten it; if the skin is moist, dry it; if the skin has no oil, oil it; if the skin shows evidence of attack by any of the itch-producing agents or organisms, protect the skin against them."   (S-24)

Scabies—the misnamed "seven-year itch"

Scabies, caused by a tiny parasitic mite that gets under the skin, tends to occur in epidemics at about fifteen-year intervals (although it was long thought to do so at seven-year intervals), and, currently, has been reported to be on the increase.

It is usually easy for a physician to diagnose in adults but in infants and children it may be mistaken for other problems unless the physician is wary.

Curative treatment is available. It may, Dr. Samuel F. Bean of Baylor College of Medicine, Houston, advises, include a prolonged hot bath and application of either gamma benzene hexachloride lotion, 25 percent benzyl benzoate emulsion, or a lotion containing benzocaine and benzyl benzoate. The medication is applied from the neck down. Usually, a second application the next morning is prescribed.   (S-25)

Ether for fever blisters

A nuisance any time they occur, fever blisters—lip sores that begin with burning and itching, then become yellowish and crusted—are recurring problems for many people. They are caused by a virus, herpes simplex, and no drug has been of any practical value.

Recently, however, two separate medical reports, one American and one from New Delhi, India, have indicated that ether, the volatile liquid that has been used for anesthesia, is of value.

A team of Indian dermatologists, testing the idea in eleven patients, tried pressing ether-laden pads directly onto fever blisters for five minutes on two consecutive days. All pain, they report, was gone within one to two minutes, and the blisters dried up within twenty-four hours and healed completely in forty-eight hours. Follow-up of the patients, they also report, found that four of the eleven had no recurrences; of the others, three had attacks separated by longer intervals than in the past.   (S-26)

Here, in the United States, Drs. G. R. Nugent and S. M. Chou of West Virginia University Medical Center, Morgantown, are using for their patients an applicator stick soaked in ether, dabbed onto a developing blister ten times, with the applications repeated three times a day. They report that blister development stops and healing starts immediately.

They also report that one of them who, for thirty-five years, regularly had three to five fever blister eruptions a year has had no eruption go beyond early stages since starting to use the ether applications and has experienced no eruptions at all more recently. They have some hope that the ether not only aborts outbreaks but may permanently eliminate the viruses residing in the lip area.   (S-27)

Psoriasis: newer treatments

A chronic, recurrent disease marked by bright red patches covered with silvery scales, psoriasis most often affects the knees, elbows, and scalp. The chest, abdomen, backs of arms and legs, palms of hands, and soles of feet are other frequently affected sites.

The cause is unknown although the fact that it seems to occur in families with a previous history of the problem suggests a hereditary factor.

Many treatments have been used. Topical corticosteroids, or cortisonelike drugs—particularly fluocinolone acetonide, flurandrenolide, and triamcinolone acetonide—have taken the place of many previous local treatments. They are usually more effective if covered with a plastic film following use at bedtime. Injections of triamcinolone acetonide directly into small, localized psoriatic lesions sometimes are used.

Other treatments have included a tar-sulfur-salicylic acid combination for the scalp, anthralin ointment applied once a day to body outbreaks, and various forms of tar, including colorless tar distillate preparations.

Often effective but usually requiring hospitalization is a system of treatment known as the Goeckerman regimen. Nightly, crude coal tar ointment is rubbed thoroughly into all affected areas except the scalp, then removed with mineral oil in the morning. The lesions are exposed daily to sunlight or ultraviolet radiation, which is increased gradually to the point of producing mild reddening of the skin. In many cases, marked improvement occurs in ten to fourteen days.

In recent years, for very severe and extensive psoriasis, methotrexate has come into use. It is given by mouth and, because it can be extremely toxic, has to be used carefully.

About half a dozen years ago, Drs. Eugene M. Farber and David E. Harris of Stanford University School of Medicine, Stanford, California, reported on using a modified form of the stiff anthralin paste often employed in the past. The new paste, somewhat like peanut butter in consistency, they found, produces less irritation and staining and allows even seriously affected patients to treat themselves at home after treatment is started in a hospital.

In the first fifty patients, forty-seven experienced clearance of psoriasis with treatment in the hospital. They then continued treatment at home, using the paste overnight three times a week, then at less frequent intervals. A follow-up of thirty-six of the patients after two to seven months of home treatment found twenty-eight without recurrences or with good control of the disease.   (S-28)

More recently, at the Letterman Army Institute of Research, Drs. Isaac Willis, now of Johns Hopkins University School of Medicine, Baltimore, and David R. Harris, now with the Veterans Administration Hospital, Palo Alto, California, tried applying a low-strength paste of anthralin, then a solution of methoxsalen, followed by black light to photoactivate the methoxsalen. Their patients were a group of men, all with chronic psoriasis that had failed to respond to usual treatment. Complete clearing of psoriasis was obtained within one to three weeks, with the clearing continuing with only occasional repeat treatments.   (S-29)

The newest treatment, one with considerable promise for the near future though still experimental, is based on an ancient Egyptian practice. The early Egyptians treated some skin diseases with some success by swallowing a powder made from a local plant and exposing themselves to sunlight.

Methoxsalen is a drug extracted from the Egyptian plant. In the new treatment, its use is coupled with exposure to high-intensity ultraviolet light produced by a special light device designed by GTE Sylvania's Light Therapy Center in Danvers, Massachusetts, and available, as of this writing, only for experimental studies going on in Boston at the Massachusetts General Hospital, in Vienna at the Allgemeines Krankenhaus, and elsewhere.

About two hours after taking methoxsalen pills, the patient either lies on a bed or is slid under a horizontal arch lined with ultraviolet light tubes, or stands in a cylindrical chamber somewhat like a shower stall, for eight to thirty minutes, depending upon the individual case.

In all of the first fifty patients treated in Boston, psoriasis was relieved completely after about a dozen sessions. Similar results have been obtained in the first eighty-five patients treated in Vienna.

How does the treatment work? The cells in psoriasis patches multiply as much as ten times faster than do normal cells. The combination of methoxsalen and extraordinary high-intensity ultraviolet light apparently slows down the multiplication process and prevents scales from forming.

More testing is needed before the treatment can be considered completely safe. More research is also needed to determine whether patients will be able to discontinue treatment. Several who, for one reason or other, could not continue with treatment have remained clear of psoriasis for as long as six months. Others who stopped treatment have had only mild recurrences.

An effective sun screen

Skin cancer, the most common malignancy in the United States, hits more than 300,000 Americans yearly, and recent studies have established that in most cases the cause is almost entirely excessive exposure to the sun. Even when it does not cause skin cancer, overexposure may cause acute skin damage and some premalignant changes that can be more painful and disfiguring than cancer itself. Additionally, constant excessive exposure to the sun has been found to multiply wrinkles and toughen the skin.

The most effective sun-screening agent available, a recent report notes, is PABA (para-aminobenzoic acid), proved to be so in both laboratory tests and outdoor trials.

PABA is available in some preparations—among them, Eclipse Sunscreen Lotion and Presun Lotion—that prevent sunburn and permit tanning, filtering out the burning rays, and helping to minimize other harmful effects such as skin cancer and premature skin aging.   (S-30)

For the super sun-sensitive

Some people are so exquisitely sensitive to sunlight that they have had to spend much of their lives sheltered from it.

They have a disorder—erythropoietic protoporphyria (EPP)—that doesn't allow them to properly handle or metabolize porphyrin, a natural body chemical. After even a few minutes' exposure to sunlight, the excess porphyrin in their skin is turned into a poisonous agent that causes itching, burning, and swelling.

Now a successful treatment has been reported by a group of investigators headed by Dr. Micheline M. Matthews-Roth of Harvard Medical School, Boston. It promises to give many EPP victims their time in the sun.

The treatment: 30-milligram doses of beta-carotene, a yellow pigment found in yellow and green leafy vegetables and yellow fruit.

Not a light filter and of no use for normal people sensitive only to sunburning radiation, carotene seems to be specific for EPP victims, acting to prevent light-exposed porphyrin from causing trouble.

In first studies with fifty-three patients, forty-six had a fourfold or greater increase in the time they could tolerate exposure to sunlight without discomfort and three others experienced a doubling in comfortable exposure time. Most of the patients now can engage in outdoor activities impossible before, and some report developing a suntan for the first time in their lives.

All told, in the first 135 patients treated, only five have not been helped. And in six years since tests first began, no side effects have been noted.

Caution the investigators: Sun-sensitive people should not try to treat themselves with carotene-containing vegetables. Several pounds a day would be needed to get the required amount of carotene for protection and such quantities could cause undesirable effects.   (S-31)

Combatting canker sores

Acute painful ulcers on the mucous membranes of the mouth, occurring singly or in groups, bother many people, in some cases as often as monthly.

The cause is still not known. For a long time, the herpes simplex virus, responsible for fever blisters, was believed to be involved, but there has been no conclusive evidence that it is. More recently, as Dr. Richard L. Zuehlke, University of Iowa, has reported, some evidence has been developed that some forms of a bacterium, the alpha-streptococcus, may be responsible.

The latter development has led to use of antibiotic syrups (notably tetracycline hydrochloride syrups) with some success.

A common regimen is to have the patient hold a teaspoonful of tetracycline hydrochloride syrup (250 milligrams per 5 cubic centimeters) on the sore or sores for five minutes before swallowing it, repeated four times a day.   (S-32)

Tinea cruris: a fungal infection

Affecting the thighs and genital area, producing burning, itching, and pain, tinea cruris often tends to recur. A newer, broad-spectrum topical agent, active against many fungi, yeasts, and bacteria, is reported to be notably effective for the problem.

In a study at the USAF Medical Center, Keesler Air Force Base, Biloxi, Mississippi, the compound—miconazole nitrate (MicaTin Cream)—freed 93.3 percent of a group of patients of signs and symptoms of the infection, often eliminating the burning, itching, and pain within twenty-four hours. Only one patient experienced a recurrence of the disease in the month after treatment was stopped. (S-33)

Warts: newer treatments

Can hypnosis be used to remove warts? So it was suggested even fifty years ago, but well-documented evidence has been lacking. Recently, a controlled study at Massachusetts General Hospital, Boston, concluded that "warts do tend to respond to hypnosis."

Seventeen patients with an average of thirty warts each were treated hypnotically once a week for five weeks and were told under hypnosis that warts on one side of the body (chosen by the patient) would soon disappear. Seven other patients, serving for comparison, received no hypnosis. Three months later, both groups were examined.

Of those hypnotized, nine, or 53 percent, showed marked improvement. A sudden loss of all warts occurred in four of the nine, gradual fading in four, and one experienced successive sudden loss of individual warts. None of the seven non-hypnotized patients showed improvement. Of these, four subsequently received hypnotherapy and three showed improvement.   (S-34)

Since warts are virus-caused, can the body's immune system—its protective mechanism against foreign invaders—be made to throw them off if stimulated?

A chemical, DNCB, is known to have such an immune stimulating effect. At the University of California, Los Angeles, School of Medicine, Dr. J. H. Greenberg and other investigators applied DNCB to some of the multiple warts on five patients. In four cases, the warts disappeared and, in two of the four, after several weeks, all the nontreated warts also vanished.   (S-35)

Vitamin A acid, valuable for acne, also has proved to be useful for people with flat warts too numerous for freezing or other usual treatment. Dr. Richard L. Zuehlke of the University of Iowa College of Medicine has reported using an 0.05 percent solution of vitamin A acid, also known as tretinoin, twice daily with good results.

For difficult-to-treat plantar warts on the soles of the feet, including the mosaic type, another preparation—glutaraldehyde in a 25 percent solution—is effective, Dr. Zuehlke also reports. Applied daily, it hardens the warts, making them easy for the patient or a family member to pare, and usually results in cure within three months.

(S-36)

CHAPTER 18

Sleep

Sleepers—the differences between long and short

Sleep requirement varies considerably. It has been estimated in various British and American studies that mean sleep time in a young adult population is about seven and three-quarter hours, with 5 percent to 10 percent sleeping over nine or under six hours in every twenty-four. But there are no adequate data for the population as a whole.

Studying the psychological characteristics of men in the two extreme groups—getting along well on either under six hours or more than nine hours—Dr. Ernest Hartman and other investigators at the Sleep Laboratory of the Boston State Hospital turned up marked differences.

Typically, the man who sleeps fewer than six hours is likely to be smooth and efficient, a hard worker, extroverted, self-assured, decisive, socially adept, ambitious, content with himself and his life, spending little time in worry, often avoiding problems by keeping busy and denying they exist.

On the other hand, the man regularly needing more than nine hours sleep tends to be a non-conformist, opinionated on many subjects, critical of society and politics, given to being something of a chronic worrier, and somewhat insecure. He may be overtly anxious, nonaggressive, somewhat inhibited sexually, not sure of the wisdom of his career choice or life-style.   (SL-1)

Lost sleep and working efficiency

How long can one go without sleep without losing much working efficiency? And how much sleep is required for recovering efficiency?

At the University of Louisville's Performance Research Laboratory investigators have found that with thirty-six hours of continuous work and loss of sleep, efficiency declines by about 15 percent; with forty-four hours, 20 percent; and with forty-eight hours, 35 percent.

They have also found that after thirty-six hours of continuous work, two hours of sleep produces 58 percent recovery of efficiency; four hours, 73 percent; and twelve hours, full recovery.   (SL-2)

New insights into insomnia and treating it

Insomnia seems to be one of the most common afflictions. According to some surveys, about half of all Americans over fifteen years of age have complained about sleeplessness at some time in their lives, about 15 percent say they experience chronic sleeping difficulty, another one-third have more or less recurrent episodes of insomnia.   (SL-2)

In an effort to find out more about the sleep of insomniacs and how it differs from the sleep of others, Dr. Ismet Karacan and other investigators at the University of Florida's sleep laboratories carried out an EEG (electroencephalogram) study with ten chronic insomniacs—eight men and two women, aged thirty to fifty-five—and ten other people, matched for age and sex, each of whom spent several nights in the laboratory, allowed to go to bed and get up in the morning as they pleased.

The overall picture for the insomniacs: they took longer to fall asleep, slept a shorter length of time, lay in bed awake longer in the morning than the others.

Other findings: Although it was expected that the insomniacs would experience much more wakefulness during the night, it turned out instead that there was no difference between the two groups in amount of time spent awake after once getting to sleep. It appears that while normal sleepers have no recollection of brief awakening periods during the night, insomniacs who have difficulty getting to sleep or who awaken early in the morning, remember the loss of sleep well.

Insomniacs also experienced more dream sleep than the others. The intervals between episodes of dream sleep for the insomniacs averaged fifty-eight minutes versus sixty-nine minutes in the others. Insomniacs also took longer to get into deep-sleep stages—sixty minutes as against twenty-nine minutes for the normal sleepers—and often obtained less deep sleep.   (SL-3)

Sleeping pills. In 1973, some five million prescriptions were filled for just one of the more popular of the thirty or so kinds of sleeping preparations physicians can prescribe.

Recent studies indicate that continued use of many of the most widely prescribed pills may only make matters worse.

Although there has been some uncertainty about whether "hangover" effects of sleeping pills are real or imagined, a careful study at London's Institute of Psychiatry has determined that such effects occur even in patients not especially aware of them.

Twelve and eighteen hours after using sleeping tablets, subjects were given reaction time and other tests for mental functioning. Definite impairment of functioning could be detected in all subjects regardless of the type of sleeping tablets used. And although many subjects thought that the tablets "generally improved" the quality of sleep and had not diminished their alertness when awake, the study found that they were simply unaware of their impaired performance.   (SL-4)

Beyond their hangover effects, sleeping pills soon lose their sleep-inducing efficacy and may actually impair sleep.

In a recent sleep laboratory study by Dr. Anthony Kales and other investigators at Pennsylvania State University, the sleep patterns of ten patients who had been taking sleeping tablets for periods ranging from months to years and despite continued use of the drugs suffered from persistent insomnia were checked as they continued to use the drugs. Their patterns were compared to those of fifteen other insomniacs who were not taking drugs.

The drug users turned out to have significantly more disturbed sleep patterns than did the others taking no medication. The pill users had fewer periods of sleep characterized by side-to-side rapid eye movement (REM) which researchers associated with dreaming. Also, drug users had as much or even more difficulty falling asleep or staying asleep and all told had longer periods of wake time.

A phenomenon associated with chronic sleeping-pill use—"drug-withdrawal insomnia"—accounts for continued use. Upon attempting to suddenly stop using pills, the insomniac experiences an increase in disturbed sleep, more frequent and intense dreams, and nightmares.

In advice to physicians about how to help patients with the phenomenon, researchers urge that the drug be withdrawn gradually at a rate of one dose every five or six days; that the patient be informed that severe changes may occur, including increased dreaming and even nightmares, and that these undesirable effects will be transient; and that, if absolutely necessary, where total withdrawal of the drug is difficult, it be replaced with flurazepam hydrochloride, a pill effective in inducing and maintaining sleep without soon losing its effectiveness.   (SL-5)

"Misuse of the bed" and learning how to fall asleep. Sleep research is a relatively new area. Many aspects of sleep remain to be investigated. One that is beginning to receive attention is the relationship between insomnia and bad sleeping habits and how such habits can be corrected.

A leader in such research is Dr. Richard R. Bootzin, a psychologist at Northwestern University, Evanston, Illinois, who considers misuse of the bed to be an especially pernicious habit.

To overcome the habit, Bootzin gives patients specific instructions as illustrated in the case of a twenty-five-year-old married man who for more than four years had gone to bed nightly at midnight and had been unable to get to sleep until three or four o'clock in the morning, stewing about job and financial problems to the point where he often turned on TV to try to stop stewing.

Bootzin's prescription for him: Go to bed only when you're tired. Once in the bedroom, no TV watching, reading, or worrying. Stay in bed to sleep, not to stew. If sleep doesn't come within a short time, leave the bed and leave the room. Return to bed only when you're ready to try to fall asleep again. And if you still don't fall asleep soon, get out of bed and out of the room again, and keep repeating the process until you do get to sleep quickly after getting back to bed. No matter if it is weekdays or weekends and no matter how much sleep you get in a night, set the alarm for the same time every morning. The body needs rest and a regular schedule will help you to get it.

Typically, the patient in this case at first had to leave the bedroom four and five times a night. But after two weeks of increasingly associating the bedroom with sleep rather than worry, reading, or TV viewing, he was getting two to four hours more sleep each night and at the end of two months was leaving the bedroom no more than once a week. (SL-6)

"Nature's sleeping pill?" A natural chemical substance that provides insomniacs with more restful sleep than drugs now being prescribed appears to have been found.

The substance: an amino acid, L-tryptophan, one of the building blocks of protein.

For some years, investigators—notably, Dr. Ernest Hartmann of Boston State Hospital—have considered that there might be some "natural hypnotic substance" used by the body in producing and regulating sleep.

Such a substance would have to be one readily available to the body either from food or through natural body synthesis processes; it should be shown to produce a normal night of sleep by scientific measurement, and to act at doses or concentrations equivalent to those that might occur naturally.

L-tryptophan, a naturally occurring amino acid, of which 0.5 to 2 grams are consumed daily in a normal diet, appears to fulfill the criteria.

In various experimental studies with men, the most common side effect of L-tryptophan proved to be drowsiness.

And in sleep laboratory studies with subjects who at home required fifteen minutes or more before they could fall asleep, Dr. Hartmann found that a dose of 1 gram of L-tryptophan halved the fall-asleep time. Moreover, thorough checking—all-night records of stages of sleep, percents, cycle length, and number of awakenings—showed that L-tryptophan produced normal-appearing sleep.

Some other intriguing possibilities exist. L-tryptophan could play a role, Dr. Hartmann suggests, in drowsiness after eating; the usual explanation that "blood leaves the head and goes to the gut" has never been very sound. Also, he notes, "the ancient prescription of a glass or two of milk at bedtime may involve more than a psychological 'association to mother.' " For the fact is that L-tryptophan is present in milk, and in other foods such as meat and green vegetables. (SL-7)

More recently, too, to test the theory that L-tryptophan may act as a natural sedative, Dr. Clinton Brown of Johns Hopkins and Dr. Althea M. I. Wagman of the Maryland Psychiatric Research Center in Catonsville, Maryland, chose twelve insomniacs who often spent up to an hour in getting to sleep. Over a two-week period, they reported to the center in Catonsville where their sleep patterns could be electronically monitored. Before going to bed, they received tablets of L-tryptophan or an inert placebo.

The study showed that the insomniacs fell asleep twice as fast with L-tryptophan as without it, and slept about forty-five minutes longer than usual without any disturbance in normal stages of sleep.

Dr. Wagman foresees the possibility of early marketing of L-tryptophan as a sleeping pill. She also points out, as does Dr. Hartmann, that the traditional home remedy for sleeplessness, a glass of warm milk, contains L-tryptophan.   (SL-8)

Bedcovers over the head: a certain risk

Many of us occasionally may pull bedcovers over the head before going to sleep. Surprisingly, however, about 11 percent of people do this regularly—and for some the practice may involve risks.

Studying healthy volunteers, investigators at the United States Army Research Institute of Environmental Medicine, Natick, Massachusetts, found that with the head covered, oxygen concentration declines by 20 percent or more and the carbon dioxide concentration is multiplied tenfold.

Such changes appear to be of no consequence for healthy adults but, the investigators warn, they may be risky for people with congestive heart failure or other conditions that allow only marginal oxygen delivery to body tissues; and excess carbon dioxide could be harmful for some who happen to be sensitive to it and who may develop abnormal heart rhythms as a result.   (SL-9)

Sleeping with open windows: healthful or old wives' tale?

Answering just that question from a physician, Dr. Donald A. Dukelow, assistant director of the American Medical Association

Department of Health Education, recently had this report to make:

Some people prefer to sleep cold; others, warm. Some are disturbed by even a slight movement of air while others prefer breezes through the bedroom. Sleeping patterns vary considerably, and what is acceptable comfort for one will be rejected by another.

But many arguments might be offered in favor of not keeping windows open in very cold weather. During sleep, many body functions diminish: body temperature falls, the heart beats more slowly, blood pressure and pulse rate fall, breathing is slower, nearly all gland secretions decrease. To add to this in midwinter the severe temperature of outdoor air adds to the body problem of maintaining reasonable temperature during sleep.

Another factor is humidity. When air temperature is below freezing, even high relative humidity represents a small amount of water vapor in the air. As the cold air enters from outside, the relative humidity of the warmed air falls below the comfort level of the breathing passages. If it is necessary to air a room, the airing should be done in the daytime to provide opportunity for the relative humidity to climb back to the comfort level before bedtime.

Sums up Dr. Dukelow:

The consensus appears to be that sleep conditions are more or less individually determined; however, the greatest comfort for most people during sleep is found when they sleep in rooms of moderate temperature and acceptable humidity, free of contaminants commonly found in the polluted atmosphere of our cities. Generally this can be obtained by not admitting very cold winter air into the sleeping room during the sleeping period.   (SL-10)

Help for nightmares and sleepwalking

Many drugs first found valuable for one specific problem turn out eventually to be useful for others.

One such drug is imipramine, first used to combat mental depression. It was subsequently found valuable in helping to control bedwetting in children.

Now Dr. Leon Tec of the Mid-Fairfield Child Guidance Center, Norwalk, Connecticut, reports its usefulness for people who experience nightmares and walk in their sleep.

In a study with a group of twelve sleepwalking and nightmare-experience children, 25 to 50 milligrams of the drug before bedtime proved effective. The compound, Dr. Tec has determined, also benefits adults with the same problems—and in both children and adults usually just two weeks of treatment is enough, and medication is not needed thereafter.   (SL-11)

CHAPTER 19

Other Problems, Other Developments

Airplane ankle

For many people, a long airplane flight means swelling of the ankles. The cause, a British investigator reports, seems to be prolonged, unrelieved bending of the knee, which may allow blood to pool in the legs and, because of the reduced circulation, permit fluid to accumulate in tissues, leading to edema with ankle swelling. Under normal circumstances, the movement of leg muscles effects a pumpinglike action that aids in moving blood upward from the legs and back to the heart. Even the relatively little leg muscle movement carried out while riding in a train or car seems enough to maintain circulation, reports Dr. H. D. Johnson of the Royal Postgraduate Medical School, London. His suggestion for airplane ankle sufferers: exercise at least the toes and ankles briefly every half hour while on a plane.   (OP-1)

Athletic injuries: heat or cold?

Even among physicians, there has been some confusion about whether to apply heat or cold for such injuries as contusions, ligament sprains, muscle strains, and fractures.

Cold, by all means, is the treatment of choice; early use of heat may, in fact, have adverse effects, reports a team of physicians and physical therapists of the Milton S. Hershey Medical Center, Hershey, Pennsylvania.

The application of ice controls edema, or swelling, and hemorrhage, and can be an important factor in rehabilitation and return of the patient to activity.

With cold, blood vessels constrict, then later dilate again. The constriction diminishes hemorrhage through damaged capillaries in the injury area. And with cold, metabolic processes within damaged cells slow down, diminishing need for oxygen and nutrients carried in the blood, and the reduction of metabolism reduces the production of edema.

With heat, on the other hand, both blood flow and metabolic rate are increased, increasing inflammation and edema, both undesirable responses.

Whatever the type of injury, the team reports, ice should be applied immediately, with the ice pack held in place with an elastic bandage wrap for a minimum of thirty minutes.   (OP-2)

Bite wounds

If the experience of one hospital emergency room is typical, bite wounds are surprisingly common, accounting for almost 1 percent of patient visits.

While dog bites are most frequent—with human and cat bites following next—dog bites tend to be more superficial, less troublesome, with a low rate of infection (a bit more than 3 percent). On the other hand, in the experience of that emergency room (Wellesley Hospital, Toronto), the infection rate in human and cat bites is almost ten times as high (30 percent).

Advises the physician in charge of the emergency room: All human and cat as well as dog bites should be treated by a physician. The human bites and cat bites deserve thorough cleansing, which may include use of saline irrigation and possibly hydrogen peroxide irrigation as well, followed by antibiotic treatment, preferably with a combination of sodium cloxacillin and either penicillin or ampicillin.

(OP- 3)

Another study indicates that as many as half of healthy dogs and even more healthy cats carry in their mouths Pasteurella Multicoda, an organism that may cause infection in a child or adult who is bitten or scratched. And often, the ten-year study at the Oregon State Public Health Laboratory indicates, the nature and cause of infection—which involves inflammation, pain, and swelling at the site of the bite or scratch, developing sometime in the next forty-eight hours—are not recognized. The infection responds to penicillin and some other antibiotics. (OP-4)

Cat scratch disease

Cats transmit it without themselves being affected. And although cat scratch disease disappears spontaneously within one to two months, it can, if not recognized for what it is, be worrisome, lead to costly medical tests, even including removal of the disease-caused lump because of suspicion of cancer.

In a little less than half the cases, the lump occurs in the neck; in the remainder it is in an arm or leg. Along with the lump, there may be malaise, headache, slight fever.

A problem with the disease is that it can result from a slight and playful scratch, symptoms do not appear until ten or more days later, and a victim has to make an effort to recall being scratched (but when they try, about 90 percent of victims can recall the incident). Laboratory tests—showing a high blood-sedimentation rate and increased gamma globulin in the blood—are helpful. So is a positive reaction to a special skin test (Frei antigen), reports Dr. Stuart Landa of the University of Chicago's Pritzker School of Medicine.   (OP-5)

A promising new treatment for Cushing's disease

Cushing's disease is the result of the release of excessive amounts of hormones by the adrenal glands atop the kidney. Symptoms of the disease may include rounded "moon" face, obesity, muscle weakness and muscle wasting, menstrual irregularities, easy bruising, and psychiatric disturbances.

A first report of striking results with a simple treatment—use of cyproheptadine, a drug commonly employed in hay fever, hives, and other allergic states—comes from Drs. Dorothy T. Krieger, Louis Amorosa, and Frederica Linica of Mount Sinai School of Medicine, New York City.

Tried in three women with Cushing's disease—two in their early thirties and the third aged forty-two—24 milligrams of the drug per day brought prompt and sustained improvement in symptoms along with reduction of the excessive hormone release.   (OP-6)

Dental developments

Remodeling discolored crowns. A quick, less expensive method of remodeling old, discolored crowns has been reported by Dr. J. D. Cox of the College of Medicine and Dentistry of New Jersey. With new plastic veneers and a powder mix applied directly to the surface of gold or acrylic crowns, the remodeling can be accomplished in many cases in a half hour appointment, and the result is said to be attractive-looking teeth.   (OP-7)

Simpler repairs of fractured teeth. A special plastic adhesive-sealant has been used to cover the biting surfaces of children's teeth and protect those vulnerable surfaces from decay. Now the same adhesive-sealant is used in a new technique for repairing fractured front teeth in children or adults without need for anesthesia or retention pins to hold the filling material in place. The adhesive-sealant is applied as a thin film over a broken tooth, a filling material is placed over the adhesive and shaped like the original tooth, and the material is hardened in two to three minutes under long-wave ultraviolet light, reports Dr. Jorge Davila of the Eastman Dental Center, Rochester, New York.   (OP-8)

Restoring the knocked-out tooth. Often now, a knocked-out tooth, child's or adult's, can be reimplanted provided certain conditions are met.

Timing is a major condition: If the tooth can be set back in place within half an hour, it very often can be saved. Even beyond that, for periods of up to six hours, there is a fair chance that interior pulp and outer periodontal tissues may survive and permit successful reimplantation.

Keeping the tooth moist until the patient can reach a dentist is another major condition.

Suggestions from dental authorities: Wrap a knocked-out tooth in a cloth wetted in water to which a little salt has been added, and get to a dentist as fast as possible.

If there is going to be a delay, try placing the tooth in the socket yourself or, if that can't be done, put it in a container of water until help can be obtained.   (OP-9)

To combat periodontal disease. Periodontal, or gum, disease involves inflammation of the gums which, over a period of time, can lead to bone loss and loosening of the teeth for lack of adequate supporting bone. The disease is a major cause of tooth loss in adults.

Promising preliminary reports suggest that vitamin E may possibly be of use in combatting the inflammation of periodontal disease, and dietary supplements of calcium may have value in increasing bone density.

At the University of California Dental School, Dr. Jo Max Goodson determined that patients with periodontal disease have in their tissues ten times the normal levels of a prostaglandin, a hormonelike body chemical capable of increasing inflammation and causing bone dissolution.

Vitamin E has some ability to inhibit prostaglandin formation. In a study with two groups of periodontal disease patients, one group received a daily dose of 800 milligrams of vitamin E with instructions to bite the capsule and swish the contents around in the mouth before swallowing so that hopefully the vitamin might have a local as well as systemic effect. The other group, for comparison, received inert capsules. After three weeks, Dr. Goodson could report, the vitamin appeared to have a definite effect in reducing inflammation, and further studies seem in order to determine whether it may control bone loss.   (OP-10)

Meanwhile, at the Graduate School of Nutrition, Cornell University, Ithaca, New York, Dr. Leo Lutwak and other investigators have been studying the possible value of calcium for bone loss. They report that in eighty periodontal disease patients treated for up to twelve months with 1,000 milligrams of calcium a day in any one of three forms—fat-free dried milk, dicalcium phosphate, or calcium gluconolactate-calcium carbonate—marked increases in lower jaw bone density have been observed.   (OP-11)

Diabetes complications

Leg artery disease. Disease of leg arteries, leading to pain on walking and in especially severe cases to pain at rest, ulceration, infection, or gangrene, may occur in diabetics and nondiabetics.

Often, for nondiabetics, surgery to bypass a damaged section of an artery has been used successfully. The same surgery has proved only slightly less successful for diabetics, report Dr. F. A. Rechle and other surgeons of the Temple University Health Sciences Center, Philadelphia, after a study with 364 patients, 46 percent of them diabetic, undergoing surgery for bypass rather than amputation.

With one type of bypass, called femorotibial, the success rate was 78 percent for nondiabetics, 60 percent for diabetics. With another, femoropopliteal, the success rate was 90 percent for nondiabetics, 82 percent for diabetics. And follow-up studies ranging from one to eleven years indicate that the bypasses continue to function well over extended periods in diabetics as well as nondiabetics.   (OP-12)

Light beams for sight-threatening diabetic retinopathy. Diabetic retinopathy, a leading cause of blindness, threatens the sight of an estimated three hundred thousand persons in the United States.

In the disease, which is associated with long-standing diabetes, new abnormal blood vessels form on the surface of the retina, the light-sensitive area at the back of the eye. The vessels may protrude into the gel-like vitreous fluid that fills the center of the eye. The vessels sometimes bleed, and although the blood may clear from the eye on its own, it often remains, causing severe loss of vision and sometimes blindness. Scar tissue also may form and then contract, resulting in detachment of the retina and blindness.

For more than a decade some physicians have used photocoagulation as a treatment for diabetic retinopathy. In photocoagulation, finely focused beams of intensive light are used to create minute burns on the retina in order to destroy or inhibit the growth of the abnormal retinal blood vessels in hope of preventing bleeding and subsequent visual loss.

One of the pioneers in the field has been Dr. Francis A. L'Esperance of Columbia-Presbyterian Medical Center, New York City. In 1973, he could report that small bursts of intense blue-green light from an argon laser were showing great promise, with treated eyes having six to ten times fewer hemorrhages on the average and far better vision than untreated eyes or unsuccessfully treated eyes (since photocoagulation is not invariably effective).

In 1976, evidence from a nationwide National Eye Institute-funded Diabetic Retinopathy Study indicated that photocoagulation can substantially reduce the risk of blindness from the disease. The evidence comes from analysis of data collected for more than two years in what will be a ten-year-long investigation going on in sixteen medical centers.

Both the green argon laser and the white xenon arc-light beams have been used. The study to date shows that photocoagulation reduces by more than half the risk of blindness in eyes with extensive new blood vessels on or near the optic disc, the place where the optic nerve meets the retina. It also indicates that treatment can reduce the risk of blindness for eyes that have hemorrhage in the vitreous fluid and either early new vessels on or near the optic disc or extensive new vessels away from the optic disc.   (OP-13)

Familial Mediterranean fever: help at last

Its cause unknown, familial Mediterranean fever has long defied treatment. The disorder produces monthly attacks of fever and severe abdominal pain. In addition, depression, drug addiction, and underachievement have been common consequences.

Varied treatments, including low-fat diets, corticosteroid drugs, other hormone therapy, psychotherapy, and more have been tried and, in some cases, even gallbladder removal, all without significant benefits.

Now, an ancient drug, one long used for gout, has proved effective. How it works is a mystery but among the first patients to be treated, a series of eleven at Massachusetts General Hospital, Boston, attacks have been strikingly reduced and in some cases eliminated. Every patient has reported dramatic improvement in life-style, with some able to resume gainful employment after previously being unable to hold jobs because of the frequency and severity of their attacks.

The drug's value has been confirmed in trials at the National Institutes of Health and abroad. And, because the drug, colchicine, is so strikingly effective, it may be used in all patients with recurrent unexplained abdominal pain and fever even as a means of diagnosis, avoiding in some cases the need for exploratory abdominal surgery.

An important fact also shown by recent research: the term "familial Mediterranean fever" is a misnomer; the disorder can occur sporadically rather than in families; and in people of non-Mediterranean extraction.   (OP-14)

Hangover help

Despite many efforts to find one, no panacea exists for alcohol hangover. Some possibly helpful suggestions, however, come from a neurologist who has studied the phenomenon.

The throbbing headache of hangover results from the alcohol-induced dilation of blood vessels in the head. Migraine preparations containing caffeine and ergotamine—or the caffeine in black coffee—help to relieve the headache because of a constricting effect on blood vessels.

Alcohol dehydrates the body, but trying to quench thirst and replace body fluid by drinking water may only aggravate nausea. Instead, several cups of salted beef broth taken at intervals will replace both fluid and lost minerals and help ease nausea.

Alcohol is metabolized and used up by the body at a constant rate. But fructose—a natural sugar found in honey, ripe fruits, vegetables, and extracts such as tomato juice—is helpful in speeding the metabolism of alcohol and thus speeding the departure of hangover.

Not least of all, being erect helps reduce blood vessel dilation; lying in bed does not.   (OP-15)

Relief for "restless legs" and night leg cramps

Cramps of the legs and foot muscles, awakening one from a sound sleep, is a common complaint for which until recently there has been no really effective method of prevention or treatment. Attacks may be relatively mild and infrequent or may occur several times a night, requiring use of heat and seriously interfering with sleep. Treatments such as use of muscle relaxants, calcium, or quinine have left much to be desired.

A closely related problem, "restless legs," may occur independently or in association with night leg cramps. It is an extremely uncomfortable feeling requiring continuous movement of the legs and finally the need to get up and walk about. An episode may last for several hours.

Several recent reports promise more or less simple relief for many sufferers. One suggests that caffeine may be a major factor in producing restless legs. In a study with fifty-five patients, all benefited from treatment consisting of avoiding caffeine-containing beverages and medications (often used to counteract the restless leg problem) and temporary use of a drug, diazepam, with sedative and muscle-relaxing activity—and continued to benefit when they continued to abstain from caffeine.   (OP-16)

Meanwhile, without regard to caffeine, Dr. Samuel Ayres, Jr., Emeritus Professor of Medicine at the University of California at Los Angeles, has reported on the value of vitamin E in both restless legs and night leg cramps.

Ayres, a dermatologist who ordinarily would not be concerned with such problems, was because both he and his wife were victims of leg cramps, his occurring every five or six weeks, sometimes lasting nearly half an hour, and requiring a heating pad, and his wife's occurring several times a week and often several times in a single night.

He became interested in vitamin E when, by chance, a patient being treated with the vitamin for a skin problem, remarked that since he had begun to take the vitamin he had stopped having nocturnal leg cramps, which had bothered him for many years.

When both Ayres and his wife took vitamin E with a prompt response, he began to make a hobby of muscle spasms.

Recently, Ayres has summarized his experience with vitamin E in 125 consecutive patients with nocturnal leg cramps and nine with restless legs.

Of the 125 with cramps, 103 experienced complete or almost complete relief; twenty showed a moderate to good response; only two failed to benefit. The cramps had been present for more than five years in sixty-eight patients, was considered severe in eighty-one, and occurred nightly or oftener in thirty-five.

Of the nine patients with restless legs of long duration, including two of his office employees, complete control was obtained in seven, 75 percent control in one, and 50 percent control in one.

Dr. Ayres prescribes vitamin E—in the form of d-alpha-tocopherol acetate or succinate—in doses of 400 International Units from one to four times daily before meals. Patients with hypertension or damaged hearts, or diabetics on insulin, he reports, should be started on much smaller doses. Inorganic iron should be avoided because it combines with and inactivates vitamin E—and this includes vitamins containing iron, and white bread or cereals fortified with iron. Frequent laxatives and mineral oil also are to be avoided. No undesirable side effects of vitamin E therapy have been encountered.   (OP-17)

Neck pain and television viewing

Mysterious neck pain, sometimes severe enough so that the victim thinks there must have been an accidental injury to the neck, often is the result of improper television viewing.

Improper viewing—from a reclining chair or a couch or bed with head resting on an arm, tilted against a headboard, or propped by pillows so the neck is unnaturally bent—not only can exacerbate and prolong pain if an injury has occurred but can be enough in itself to produce neck pain, reports one physician, Dr. David Goldberg, Springfield, Massachusetts.

The best treatment is simply not to watch TV in a lying-down position.   (OP-18)

Obesity

False notions and natural history. Obese people are commonly supposed to either eat more than others or to use up calories more economically and maybe have difficulty in releasing body fat for energy. But none of this is necessarily the case, Mayo Clinic investigators have found.

Studying both normal and obese people, they have determined that the obese make normal use of carbohydrates, fats, and proteins and mobilize fat for energy as readily as normal people.

They have also found that the basal metabolic rate of all people tends to decline with age so that those of normal weight can become obese all too readily as they grow older if they don't change exercise and eating habits. Even those who eat a bit less as they age may gain weight if they fail to increase physical activities. For this reason, the person who complains that "I don't eat as much as I used to but I have gained weight" may well be right.

Checking on the records of many patients seen at the clinic over a thirty-year period, the investigators found that, for example, a man who weighs 154 at age thirty and who fails to increase his exercise or cut his food intake can expect to weigh over 200 pounds by age sixty.

To remain at ideal weight from age thirty to age sixty, if exercise is not increased, men generally have to cut caloric intake by 11 percent and women by 5 percent over the thirty-year period. Adequate physical activity, the Mayo research indicates, can play an important part in consuming calories to counter the decrease in caloric needs with age.   (OP-19)

Added insights on exercise. At Georgetown University School of Medicine, Washington, D.C., a medical team studied two groups of obese patients, one following diet alone, the other coupling diet with thirty minutes of exercise a day. The exercisers showed greater weight loss, and, notably, greater loss of fat instead of lean tissue, and also a lower heart beat at rest and quicker return of heart rate to normal after activity. Both of the latter are indicative of physical fitness in general and of heart fitness in particular.   (OP-20)

Is exercise alone effective for weight reduction? At the University of California, Irvine, Dr. Grant Gwinup worked with a group of obese women who for twelve months did half an hour or more of brisk walking daily. No dietary restrictions were imposed and the women in fact ate somewhat more than before because of increased appetite from exercise. Yet they lost from ten to thirty-eight pounds—an average of twenty-two—from the brisk walking alone. To be sure, as Dr. Gwinup notes, exercise alone is no easy answer to obesity, but for some people it does provide an alternative to dieting that can cause weight loss and provide in addition other health benefits from exercise.   (OP-21)

Whether special exercises for a particular body site can melt away fat is a controversial matter. In one study, investigators at the Orange County (California) Medical Center measured the forearms of both professional and amateur tennis players. Invariably, they found, the forearm circumference in the playing arm was bigger than in the nonplaying, but the thickness of fat under the skin was virtually identical in both arms.   (OP-22)

But in another study by investigators at Cornell University and Ithaca (New York) College, sixteen women college students weighing up to 140 pounds and averaging 121 went through nine weeks of special exercises. Five times a week, while lying down, they moved their legs through fifteen revolutions, a simple isokinetic exercise. They also used an isometric exercise in which, with knees first at 90 degrees and then at 45, they contracted thigh muscles as hard as they could for five seconds for three repetitions. Although the exercises were not vigorous enough to lead to any weight loss, skinfold measurements showed a decrease of under-the-skin fat in the thighs but not elsewhere in unexercised sites.   (OP-23)

Achieving eating behavior control. Promising results have been obtained with a behavior modification approach to the obesity problem.

In one of the first studies, at the University of Pennsylvania, Philadelphia, a group of obese patients were asked to follow a few definite rules. They were to keep a daily record in detail of their eating activities to establish how much they ate, the speed of eating, and circumstances associated with eating. They were also to confine any eating, including snacking, to one place rather than, as many obese do, eat in various places at different times of the day.

Additionally, they were to use a distinctively colored place mat and napkin and to make eating a pure experience involving no other activity such as reading, watching TV, or arguing with their families. Finally, they were to count each mouthful of food during a meal and deliberately put utensils back on the plate after every third mouthful until that mouthful was thoroughly chewed and swallowed.

The obese patients in the group lost more weight than another comparable group receiving conventional group psychotherapy. More than half—53 percent—lost more than twenty pounds and 13 percent lost more than forty.   (OP-24)

In a later study at Stanford University School of Medicine, Stanford, California, a somewhat modified approach was used. Dieters participated in a weekly group therapy session and in addition were asked to keep a diary in which they entered daily what, when, and where they ate, with whom, and their emotional state while eating, the objective being to make eating less an automatic reflex action and more a conscious effort. The results: half the patients lost twenty or more pounds in ten to twenty weeks and have kept the weight off for at least a year.   (OP-25)

Help for osteoporosis

Osteoporosis, a thinning of bone structure, often causes bone pain and may also lead to loss of height, repeated bone fractures, and in very severe cases to invalidism. It tends to be particularly common in women after menopause.

One promising treatment combines calcium and fluoride supplements plus vitamin D. At Mayo Clinic, Dr. Jenifer Jowsey has found that women on the treatment have experienced improvement in symptoms and increase in bone formation. Follow-up studies have shown that those continuing on the treatment experienced no fractures at all after the first year and showed evidence of increased bone mass after three years. Furthermore, after five years the bone mass remained at the healthily increased level.   (OP-26)

At the University of California, San Francisco, in a study that began in 1948, Dr. Gilbert S. Gordan and other investigators have found that estrogen treatment is effective in stopping fractures, and the treatment apparently does not increase risk of cancer. In the 220 women who have been on estrogen treatment over the prolonged period, twenty cancers were to be expected; only eight actually occurred.   (OP-27)

In another study at the University of Washington, Seattle, Dr. Charles H. Chesnut III and other physicians have studied use of a drug, methandrostenolone (Dianabol), in thirteen osteoporotic women who received 5 milligrams a day three weeks on and one week off, while another similar group of women, for comparison, received look-alike, but inert, medication. During the two-year study, all the drug-treated women either gained calcium (which is lost in osteoporosis) or showed no significant loss of it. In contrast, the others lost calcium or showed no significant change in calcium levels. The treated women also reported some reduction of back pain.   (OP-28)

Overbreathing as a cause of many symptoms, including chest pain

Unusually prolonged and unusually deep breathing commonly accompanies anxiety and tension. It has been known to produce many worrisome symptoms—palpitation or pounding of the heart, fullness in the throat, pain over the stomach region, numbness around mouth, arms, and feet, or muscular spasm of the hands and feet.

A recent study by Dr. C. E. Wheatley of Northville, Michigan, indicates that, surprisingly often, overbreathing—also known as hyperventilation—may be responsible, with or without the presence of others of its symptoms, for chest pain that resembles the angina associated with coronary heart disease, and that failure to recognize this may lead to undue worry about and unnecessary tests for heart disease.

In the study, fifteen of ninety-five consecutive patients with chest pain turned out to have it because of hyperventilation. Reassurance and explanation of the phenomenon led to relief and, when examined again twenty-four to forty-four months later, all fifteen patients were less symptomatic.   (OP-29)

For attacks of hyperventilation symptoms, some physicians have found that rebreathing into a paper bag to replace the carbon dioxide "blown off" during hyperventilation often provides quick relief.

Paget's disease: new treatment for an old disorder

The first safe and effective treatment promises relief for severely afflicted victims of Paget's disease.

The disease, which affects an estimated 2.5 million people in the United States, 125,000 of them very severely, involves, first, abnormal thinning of bone, then followed by unregulated new bone formation. But the new bone lacks strength, has abnormal structure, and may become deformed and cause pain.

In some cases, Paget's disease is obvious. The head may become enlarged because of abnormal new bone growth; the legs may become bowed because of the bone weakness; collapse of weakened bones in the spine may produce hunching of the back.

But often the disease can be misleading. A patient may have no obvious sign but will have nonspecific symptoms such as pain, headaches, increasing deafness, ringing of the ears, or muscle or sensory disturbances from nerve compression caused by pagetic bone.

The diagnosis may not be made because of a low index of suspicion. But it is relatively simple to identify Paget's. X-rays show characteristic changes, and a simple blood test reveals an increase of an enzyme, alkaline phosphatase, in the serum.

No specific treatment has been available. Aspirin and indometha-cin, a drug sometimes employed for arthritis, have been used to help relieve pain. For more severely afflicted patients, cortisonelike agents and estrogen and androgen drugs have been tried.

The new treatment uses calcitonin, a hormone produced by the thyroid gland. Calcitonin is normally present in the blood. It is even present in the blood of Paget patients. Yet, for some reason, when it is injected in Paget patients, it seems to prevent the excessive break-down of bone characteristic of the disease.

Calcitonin for the first trials was obtained from pigs but it had relatively weak activity. Calcitonin obtained from salmon had greater strength. More recently, scientists have been able to make the hor-mone synthetically, and synthetic salmon calcitonin, now available for medical use, has great potency.

In one of the first studies at Johns Hopkins University School of Medicine, Baltimore, the synthetic material, when injected daily, proved effective within three to six weeks in 87 percent of patients. Dr. C. R. Hamilton, Jr., director of the Endocrine Research Laboratory at the United States Air Force Medical Center, Lackland Air Force Base, San Antonio, who carried out some of the first trials, has found no significant undesirable effects in patients treated thus far for three years.

Other studies have confirmed the value of calcitonin, which re-cently has received Food and Drug Administration approval. In a late report, Dr. Stanley Wallach of Albany Medical College, Albany, New York, summing up experience of many studies, indicates that benefits from synthetic salmon calcitonin can be expected in 75 percent of patients, with improvement or complete relief of pain and other symptoms often achieved as early as two weeks after the start of treatment. And although calcitonin has one disadvantage—it has to be injected—most patients can be taught to inject it subcutaneously in the thigh. The procedure is no more difficult than self-administration of insulin by diabetics.   (OP-30)

For Raynaud phenomenon: a drug treatment and biofeedback

Involving spasm of small blood vessels, Raynaud phenomenon produces intermittent episodes of blanching or blueness of fingers or toes after exposure to cold or during emotional upsets, sometimes accompanied by numbness and, as an attack wears off, by throbbing pain.

Although the problem may be associated with artery or other disease, it also appears without clear cause in young women.

Injections into an artery of a drug, reserpine, often used as a tranquilizing agent and for high blood pressure, may be helpful in many cases. In a study at Duke University Medical Center, Durham, North Carolina, two-thirds of 102 patients so treated benefited, with relief continuing in some for many months after an injection. (OP-31)

Meanwhile, an early report of a study in Boston suggests that biofeedback may have value. At Massachusetts General Hospital, Dr. Alan M. Jacobson and other physicians had as one patient a thirty-one-year-old man with long-standing Raynaud phenomenon. Hypnosis was tried but proved inadequate.

The patient then was taught to use a special temperature sensing and training device. The device produces an audible tone that changes in pitch as finger temperature is increased. In usual biofeedback training fashion, the patient, concentrating on doing anything he could possibly do to change the pitch, learned how to increase finger temperature and, thereafter, remembering how he had done so with the trainer, could begin to do so without using the machine. After eight training sensations, he was able to control finger temperature successfully enough to be able for the first time in many years to touch a cold object without experiencing pain. More than seven months later, he was still able to regulate warmth and color of both hands at will.   (OP-32)

A simple relaxation technique

A simple three-step relaxation technique requiring only a few minutes to learn has been reported by Drs. A. P. French and J. P. Tupin of the University of California, Davis, to be helpful in many cases in relieving insomnia, moderate pain and anxiety, and emotional reactions to illness.

The directions given by the physicians: Sit comfortably, feet on floor, eyes closed, and let breathing become relaxed, with air gently flowing into and out of the lungs, after which it will be easy to relax muscles.

In the second step, relax the mind, letting it drift naturally and gently to some pleasant, relaxing, restful memory. Usually, this is achieved within one minute.

In the third step, "simply present that memory very gently to your mind and allow yourself to be there and experience that memory. Don't concentrate on it or think about it in the usual sense, and if your mind wanders off simply bring yourself back, very gently and very naturally, by presenting the memory to your mind again."

In their experience, the physicians report, the technique can be learned by most people in just three or four minutes and in many cases results immediately in both relaxation and a sense of well-being.

(OP-33)

A help for sciatica

Sciatica, which has been described by some victims as a "kind of toothache in the leg," produces severe pain along the course of the sciatic nerve, frequently from buttock to foot.

In sciatica, the nerve is inflamed and, because of its position and length, the sciatic nerve is more exposed to internal and external injury and inflammation than any other nerve in the body. Joint disease such as arthritis of the hip or lumbosacral joint may sometimes give rise to sciatic nerve pain. But most often—in about 90 percent of cases—sciatica results from compression or injury of the nerve or its roots in the spine because of a disk problem or other spinal disorder such as arthritis in the spine.

A hopeful report on use of an injection of a cortisonelike drug, methylprednisolone acetate, into an irritated area of spine from which sciatic pain often may stem comes from a group of orthopedic surgeons—Drs. J. T. Hartman, now at Texas Tech University School of Medicine, A. P. Winnie and S. Ramamurthy of the University of Illinois Hospital, Chicago, and M. R. Mani and H. L. Meyers, Jr., of Cook County Hospital, Chicago.

Of thirty patients, twenty-seven experienced complete relief of pain after one or more injections into the spine (epidural). Of thirty-seven receiving injections into a sheath (intrathecal), twenty-seven were completely freed of pain and seven others experienced improvement. Of sixteen patients who received both types of injections when relief with one proved inadequate, fourteen had complete relief.   (OP-34)

Taste, smell, and the thyroid

In some patients with taste or smell disturbances, or both, the problem, it now appears, may lie with hypothyroidism, or underfunctioning of the thyroid gland.

At Saint Louis's Barnes Hospital, Dr. Robert J. McConnell, in a study of hypothyroid patients, found that half were aware of either diminished or distorted sense of taste, and one-third had both problems. Many also complained of defects in the sense of smell.

After correction of the hypothyroid condition by thyroid replacement treatment, four of every five of the patients were cured of the taste and smell disorders, the earliest in sixteen days.   (OP-35)

For smokers: a way to reduce risk

In an unusual study at the University of Louisville School of Medicine, Dr. W. H. Anderson used special monitoring equipment to establish cigarette "puff profiles" for 779 men and 154 women, forty-seven of whom had lung cancer. The profiles showed marked differences between the cancer group and other smokers.

The patients with cancer consumed much more tar, smoked each cigarette an average of one minute and twelve seconds longer, smoked more before breakfast, and their total daily smoking time, at two hours and twenty-eight minutes, was approximately twice as long as for the other smokers.

Based on the study, Dr. Anderson suggests that while eliminating cigarette smoking entirely would be best, short of that, lung cancer risk may possibly be reduced by use of cigarettes with relatively high nicotine but low tar content, limiting smoking to a maximum of one pack a day, and not permitting a cigarette to last longer than three and a half minutes to minimize total smoking exposure and tar consumption.   (OP-36)

Stitch-in-the-side with exercise

The sharp pain that may pop up in the liver or spleen area during vigorous physical activity has nothing to do with liver or spleen and does not mean that activity should be restricted.

Instead, reports Dr. Allan J. Ryan of the University of Wisconsin, Madison, such stitch-in-the-side pain stems from entrapment of gas in the colon and contractions of the colon that occur during exercise when the bowel has not been properly emptied beforehand.

If necessary, in people who are particularly susceptible, an intestinal antispasmodic medicine may be prescribed for use one to two hours before starting vigorous activity as a means of preventing the cramping.   (OP-37)

Stuttering: effective new approaches

Stuttering has often been considered to be an emotional disorder. But at the Temple University Speech Research Laboratory in Philadelphia, it is looked upon as an organic or physical predisposition problem centering in the larynx or voice box.

At the laboratory, a 90 percent success rate in ending stuttering over an average period of two to three months for adults, sometimes less for children, has been achieved with a breathing technique that teaches a "breathier, natural, softer" voice.

Instead of pursing lips together tightly, anticipating trouble before they utter a word, stutterers learn to touch their lips together softly and speak in a soft, easy tone. The softer voice changes the basic position of the larynx and in doing so short-circuits the stuttering mechanism, laboratory investigators report.

Deconditioning or desensitizing is also used to gradually build up confidence of stutterers in what is for them their most difficult, stuttering-inducing situations. Thus, for example, those terrified of the phone are encouraged first to simply think about the phone while talking with their new voices, then to practice while looking at the phone, then while touching the phone, and, finally, while actually talking into the phone.   (OP-38)

Another technique, in which the stutterer speaks in time with the regular beat of a metronome, has been under study in various laboratories for many years. Gradually, it has been refined from a laborious one-word-per-beat effort to several words per beat so speech sounds natural rather than staccato.

The metronome method is in increasing use by speech therapists. In what may be a further refinement, being used successfully at a stuttering clinic at Long Island Jewish-Hillside Medical Center, New

Hyde Park, New York, a miniature metronome, worn like a hearing aid, is employed. At weekly group sessions, stutterers learn how to adjust the tiny pacing device that helps control speech. With home practice, most stutterers, according to the clinic, show marked improvement within weeks.

One of the newest techniques, called Habit Reversal Procedure, has been reported by Drs. N. H. Azrin and R. C. Nunn, research psychologists at the Behaviour Research Laboratory, Anna (Illinois) State Hospital.

In the new procedure, a stutterer interrupts his speech at moments of actual or anticipated stuttering and at natural pause points and resumes speaking immediately after breathing deeply during the pause. In addition to the regularized pausing and breathing, the program includes other factors such as formulating thoughts prior to speaking, identifying stutter-prone situations, identifying mannerisms associated with stuttering, speaking for short durations when tense or nervous, daily breathing exercises, and relaxation procedures.

All of this, the two psychologists report, can be taught in a single counseling session of about two hours. Thereafter, over a two-week follow-up period, a counselor phones each patient daily to check progress.

Results in the first patients so treated have been striking: 94 percent reduction of stuttering on the first day, further improvement thereafter. The treatment is reported to have been effective for patients who stuttered very severely (one thousand episodes per day) as well as for those who stuttered rarely (two episodes a day) but distressingly.

(OP-39)

Tennis elbow

A painful, even disabling form of bursitis, tennis elbow is a common problem, particularly among less experienced players.

According to a study by Dr. Robert P. Nirschl, chief of orthopedic surgery at Northern Virginia Doctors Hospital, Arlington, an experienced player uses the power source of shoulder muscles as well as body weight force in swinging a racket, reducing strain on the elbow. The inexperienced player, on the other hand, usually tends to rely on the power force of the forearm, which transmits much strain to the elbow, especially in backhand strokes.

The type of racket used also is a factor. Metal rackets, particularly stainless steel alloys, Dr. Nirschl finds, tend to apply least force against the elbow when the racket is swung. He also recommends a stringing tension not greater than fifty pounds.

Another study, by Dr. James D. Priest of Stanford University Hospital, Stanford, California, suggests similarly that use of a steel or aluminum racket—and, in addition, of a two-handed rather than one-handed backhand stroke—makes for the best chance of avoiding tennis elbow.

If a player experiences immediate pain in the elbow after a game, he should apply ice over a twenty-four-hour period, advises Dr. Nirschl, and if the pain persists he should get medical help. Often tennis elbow will respond to further treatment with massage and mild heat. Severe cases may require injections of antiinflammatory drugs.   (OP-40)

After another study involving 871 tennis elbow patients, Drs. Harold B. Boyd, Emeritus Professor of Orthopedic Surgery at the University of Tennessee, Memphis, and A. C. McLeod of Hatties-burg, Mississippi, have reported that only forty did not respond to rest or injections and required surgery. Surgery, if necessary, can provide relief of pain and restoration of full motion in almost all cases, with the patient usually able to resume work and hobbies in six weeks. But three to six months are required for regaining full strength in the forearm.   (OP-41)

Water: simple disinfection

Many methods have been used by travelers, campers, hikers, and others who must use drinking water of unknown quality. But a particularly simple method that produces safe and palatable water has been reported by Drs. F. H. Kahn and B. R. Visscher of the University of California, Los Angeles.

It involves obtaining iodine crystals from a drugstore, placing four to eight grams of them in a one-ounce glass bottle, filling the bottle with water, shaking vigorously, and allowing them to settle.

When 12½ cubic centimeters of the solution is then added to a quart of water, any disease-causing organisms—bacteria, viruses, and amoeba as well—are inactivated within fifteen minutes. The iodine crystals can be used almost a thousand times to make a fresh solution.

Water disinfected this way has an acceptable taste. It can be even more palatable, the physicians report, if only 5 rather than 12½ cubic centimeters of the solution are used with a quart of water, but the waiting period then must be forty-five minutes to an hour rather than fifteen minutes.   (OP-42)

CHAPTER 20
Drugs and Drug Taking

The value of modern medicines, many of them extremely potent, is unquestionable. But if they have great potential for good, it becomes clearer each day that some, even many, have potential for harm, especially when indiscriminately used, abused, or improperly used.

What follows are among the most important recent insights that could have practical value for you or someone in your family.

Prescription confusion

When, recently, a special study was done at the University of Rochester Medical Center on how patients interpreted instructions on each of ten prescription labels, *not once* was a label uniformly interpreted by all patients.

One prescription, for example, called for taking penicillin G three times a day and at bedtime. The vast majority—89.5 percent—of

215

patients interpreted that to mean: take the drug with meals and at bedtime. But some drugs—and penicillin G is one—should be taken on an empty stomach to facilitate its absorption and effective activity.

Reported the investigators: "We discovered a surprisingly wide range of interpretations, a high frequency of misinterpretations, and a significant potential for failure or illness as a consequence of mistaken interpretations."

They urged physicians to provide better instructions on how to take medication and to review the instructions with patients.

The lesson for any patient: If a prescription label is not specific or clear enough on how and when to take the medication, don't guess; insist that the physician tell you.   (D-1)

A lot of prescriptions versus real medical attention

Not long ago, concerned about drug prescribing problems, Drs. Peter P. Lamy and Robert E. Vestal of the University of Maryland and Vanderbilt University respectively reported a case illustrative of what may be a not uncommon problem.

An elderly woman had high blood pressure, congestive heart failure, diabetes, and ankle swelling, and was obese. Her physician had prescribed a reducing diet plus an oral antidiabetes drug, plus Peritrate and nitroglycerin drugs for her heart, a thiazide diuretic for her elevated blood pressure, and antacids for her vague complaints about stomach upsets.

In all probability, Drs. Lamy and Vestal point out, only two of the drugs are justified. The diuretic is appropriate for both her congestive heart failure and high blood pressure, but it could make treatment of her diabetes more difficult. In that case, insulin instead of the oral antidiabetes drug should be considered—although, in fact, her diabetic problem might well diminish or disappear altogether if she could lose weight.

Unfortunately, the woman had not been led to understand either the diet or its importance and has not followed it. She continues to overeat and her physician treats her gastric symptoms with antacids. Both Peritrate and nitroglycerin were prescribed only because of the vague complaint that her chest hurt. Taking the diuretic only erratically, she has had little benefit from it.

"In 10 years," Drs. Lamy and Vestal note, "the physician has not changed the regimen at all, even though lack of success should have prompted review and change. It would have been far better for the physician to have taken the time to explain the need for adhering to the diet, to make sure the diuretic was taken as directed, and to consider whether the chest pains merited any drug therapy at all. Our conclusion is that in this patient drug prescribing has replaced real medical attention."   (D-2)

Named prescriptions

Should you as a patient know the names of all medications prescribed for you? Should the labels indicate the names as well as prescription number and directions?

More and more physicians now believe so. But not all instruct pharmacists to so label.

Not long ago, under the heading of "chromoconfusion," a medical report in the *Journal of the Canadian Medical Association* called attention to the problem.

Suppose, as an example, it suggested to physicians, that you are treating a man suffering from severe high blood pressure, mild anginal chest pain, hyperuricemia (elevated uric acid levels in the blood), mild diabetes, and congestive heart failure. And suppose, it also suggested, that you happen to prescribe these drugs, all of them justified for treating all aspects of the poor man's many ailments: Lanoxin, Hygroton, Isordil, Ismelin, Serpasil, Zyloprim, and D.B.I.

The prescriptions are not labeled, and these happen to be all "little white pills"—which is the only way the patient can refer to them.

"Try to envision," the Canadian report proposed, "how to ask your patient, the next time he comes to your office, how compliant he is about taking the 'little round white pill for the heart,' the 'little round white pill for water,' the 'little round white pill for blood pressure,' and the 'little round white pill for angina.' If he brings the pills with him, just think how you will be confused; if he does not bring the pills with him, just imagine your frustrating conversation about all those 'little round white pills.' Unknowingly, you have now become a little-round-white-pill doctor. And we would not be surprised if some of your clientele would not develop decompensated heart failure, digitalis intoxication, uncontrolled hypertension, orthostatic hypotension, etc."

Naming drugs on labels can be important for helping to avoid mistakes in taking medication. If undesirable side effects or serious reactions should arise during the course of taking a medication, if there should be an accidental overdose, or if a child should get hold of and use the medication, immediate identification of the compound may well help to prevent fatality. Moreover, your knowledge of what you are taking can be valuable if you have to consult another physician while on a trip or when your physician is away.

So if your drugs are not now identified on prescription labels, you may want to ask your physician to see to it that they are.   (D-3)

Drug-drug interactions

When two or more drugs are being used, each may do its job without interference with the other. Sometimes, one may even help the other.

But it is also possible for use of one drug on top of another to be harmful. One may interfere with the activity of the other, rendering it useless. Or the use of a second drug may make it necessary to reduce the dosage of the first—or raise it—to avoid harm.

Consider, for example, a patient who was hospitalized for a heart attack, recovered from it, was released from the hospital, and ten days later developed an alarming condition.

While in the hospital, he had received anticoagulant medication to prevent blood clotting as part of treatment after the heart attack. At home, he went on, as directed, taking the medication in the same dosage. But now the anticoagulant was producing excessive thinning of the blood.

Why the dangerous change? It turned out that in the hospital the patient had received phenobarbital upon retiring at night. The sedative, in the course of its handling in the body, stimulated liver chemicals that broke down the anticoagulant faster. At home, without the sedative, the anticoagulant activity continued longer and was more potent. Without the sedative, the patient was now getting in effect an overdose of anticoagulant. The problem, once understood, was quickly solved with a change in anticoagulant dosage.

Here are just a few other of many hundreds of examples of drug interaction. When a patient is taking aspirin, addition of an anticoagulant can lead to bleeding. If a patient is using an antidepressant drug such as amitriptyline and is also given guanethidine for high blood pressure, the amitriptyline nullifies the pressure-lowering activity of guanethidine. If a patient is taking an antihistamine for allergy and uses alcohol, central nervous system depression may sometimes follow.

Understanding—and taking into account—interactions between drugs is coming to be virtually a new science in medicine.

As a patient, your best protection lies in letting a physician you consult about a new condition know what if any drugs you may already be taking, both prescription drugs and ordinary over-the-counter drugs such as aspirin or other pain relievers, antacids, laxatives, and the like. It also lies in asking a physician, when he prescribes a drug, whether it will be all right, if necessary, to take aspirin or other agents.   (D-4)

Drug-diet interactions

Among the best known interactions between drugs and food is the serious, even potentially fatal interaction between certain antidepressant drugs known as MAO inhibitors—including Marplan, Parnate, Eutonyl, Nardil, and Niamid—and foods containing the compound tyramine.

Some physicians, when prescribing one of these drugs, instruct pharmacists to print on the label: "No cheese, no chicken livers."

Some deaths have been reported from interactions between MAO inhibitors and tyramine-rich foods that have led to blood pressure crises and brain hemorrhage.

Besides cheese and chicken livers, pickled herring and Chianti wine belong in the tyramine-rich group and are to be avoided by anyone using a MAO inhibitor.

Some drugs may impair food absorption; some foods may impair drug absorption. Some drugs are best taken on an empty stomach; some, at other times; and some should never be taken with some particular foods.

A recent report on drug and diet interactions offers these useful guidelines:

To be taken on an empty stomach (2 to 3 hours before meals):
benzathine penicillin G
cloxacillin (Tegophen)

erythromycin
lincomycin (Lincocin)
methacycline (Rondomycin)
phenoxymethyl penicillin (penicillin V)
tetracyclines, except demethylchlortetracycline (Declomycin)
    which can easily upset the stomach

To be taken ½ hour before meals:

belladonna and its alkaloids
chlordiazepoxide hydrochloride (Librax)
hyoscyamine sulfate (Donnatal)
methylphenidate (Ritalin)
phenazopyridine (Pyridium)
phenmetrazine hydrochloride (Preludin)
propantheline bromide (Pro-banthine)

To be taken with meals or food:

aminophylline
antidiabetics
APC (acetylsalicylic acid, phenacetin, caffeine)
chlorothiazide (Diuril, Hydrodiuril)
diphenlhydantoin (Dilantin)
mefenamic acid (Ponstel)
metronidazole (Flagyl)
nitrofurantoin (Furadantin, Macrodantin)
prednisolone
prednisone
rauwolfia and its alkaloids
reserpine (Serpasil)
triamterene (Dyrenium)
trihexyphenidyl hydrochloride (Artane)
trimeprazine tartrate (Temaril)

Not to be taken with milk:

bisacodyl (Dulcolax)
potassium chloride
potassium iodide
tetracyclines except doxycycline (Vibramycin)

Not to be taken with fruit juices:

ampicillin
benzathine penicillin G
cloxacillin (Tegopen)
erythromycin

Alcohol to be avoided while taking:

acetohexamide (Dymelor)
antihistamines
chloral hydrate
chlordiazepoxide (Librium)
chlorpropamide (Diabinese)
diphenoxylate hydrochloride (Lomotil)
MAO inhibitors (Marplan, Parnate, Eutonyl, Nardil, Niamid)
meclizine hydrochloride (Antivert)
methaqualone (Quaalude)
metronidazole (Flagyl)
narcotics
phenformin hydrochloride (DBI)
tolbutamide (Orinase)   (D-5)

Avoiding a problem with antacids

Antacids commonly contain aluminum hydroxide alone or combined with magnesium hydroxide. Recent research indicates that
such preparations may, unless precautions are taken, have harmful
effects on bones.

At the Veterans Administration Hospital, Hines, Illinois, tests in
men taking small doses of the antacids, doses much lower than often
used by ulcer patients, revealed calcium and phosphorus losses.
Losses of the two minerals over a prolonged period can produce a
softening of bone (osteomalacia) similar to that of childhood rickets.

Suggests Dr. Herta Spencer, who carried out the tests: Use of
foods such as meat and milk which contain adequate amounts of
calcium and phosphorus may be needed to prevent harmful deficien-
cies in antacid users.   (D-6)

How to take aerosol medications

Medications in aerosol form are often used to treat airway obstruction and breathing difficulties. The common practice in taking them is to close one's lips around the aerosol mouthpiece and inhale.

A possibly more effective method now is suggested by a British study. At Darlington Memorial Hospital, Darlington, England, a comparison was made in thirty-one patients of the closed-lips-inhale method and another technique in which the aerosol is held close to and aimed into the open mouth. The latter technique led to greater improvement in symptoms, a possible reason being that it involves less swallowing of the aerosol with more left to act on the breathing passages.   (D-7)

On using aspirin

A valued drug and one of the safest, aspirin nevertheless sometimes causes gastrointestinal bleeding. Some reports have indicated that in as many as one of every seven or eight patients hospitalized for a bleeding problem, aspirin is involved.

Aspirin, some studies have suggested, should always be taken with food or at least a glass of milk to minimize the likelihood of stomach irritation and bleeding.   (D-8)

A recent report by Dr. Martin I. Blake of the University of Illinois College of Pharmacy, Chicago, indicates that gastrointestinal bleeding from aspirin is the result of a local effect of aspirin particles. The report urges doctors and druggists to advise patients not to swallow aspirin tablets whole but rather to chew them thoroughly and swallow with plenty of water or, alternatively, to crush the tablets to a fine powder and take the powder in orange juice.   (D-9)

Aspirin for dental problems. Surprisingly, although codeine is commonly used to relieve moderate to severe pain after dental surgery, aspirin (and the aspirin substitute, acetaminophen) can be more effective.

In a recent study in which 160 patients—after removal of impacted third molar teeth—received either codeine, aspirin, acetaminophen, or combinations of acetaminophen or aspirin with codeine, both aspirin and acetaminophen proved more effective for the relief of pain than did codeine, and a combination of aspirin or acetaminophen with codeine was not markedly superior to aspirin or acetaminophen alone.

In addition to being less costly than codeine, the two nonnarcotic drugs allow patients to function better because of fewer side effects.   (D-10)

When it comes to relieving toothaches, aspirin can be valuable, but a tablet should never be placed on or near an aching tooth. Used that way, aspirin can produce burning and ulcerated sores and may even damage the tooth nerve or pulp. Aspirin for toothaches should be taken internally.   (D-11)

When medicines produce "Sahara" mouth

An unpleasant side effect of some antidepressant and other medications is excessive drying of the mouth, referred to by some patients as "Sahara" mouth.

One physician reports that the best way to combat the problem in his experience—and the discovery was actually made by several of his patients—is to use ice chips. They are longer-acting and often more effective than cold water, without the loading effect of large quantities of water, and are more gratifying than chewing gum or mints.   (D-12)

On nitroglycerin for heart patients

Nitroglycerin is an old, reliable, remarkably effective drug for angina pectoris, the chest pain associated with coronary heart disease. The drug not only can provide quick relief for an angina attack; when taken prior to any activity known to bring on an attack, it often can prevent the attack.

A matter of position. A very recent study shows that the best way to take nitroglycerin is while standing up.

The drug provides relief by dilating the coronary arteries so more blood and oxygen can flow through them and reach the heart muscle. It has also been suggested that the drug helps another way: by reducing the size of the heart's main pumping chamber, thus decreasing the heart muscle's need for oxygen.

And recently, at Johns Hopkins University, Baltimore, Dr. N. J. Fortuin and other investigators, using special techniques for viewing the heart chamber, have determined that in fact nitroglycerin does reduce the chamber size within three minutes after it is taken—and is more effective in doing so when it is used while standing upright. (D-13)

Fresh nitroglycerin. When nitroglycerin deteriorates with age, it loses much or all of its value.

One study by Dr. H. W. Copelan of Albert Einstein Medical Center, Philadelphia, has provided a simple means by which patients can tell for themselves when nitroglycerin is still fresh and useful. Nitroglycerin is one of the very few drugs that are best absorbed by the body when placed under the tongue. And when placed under the tongue, nitroglycerin, the study indicates, should produce a burning sensation. When it does, it is still fresh and potent; when it does not, it is likely to be of no value.   (D-14)

Another study concerned with potency loss offers useful information for patients for keeping nitroglycerin fresh and potent longer.

Carried out by Dr. G. A. Mayer of the Laboratories for Therapeutic Research, Kingston, Ontario, the study found that nitroglycerin tablets, when stored in a refrigerator in a small, amber, tightly capped glass bottle remain potent and useful for up to five months, whereas tablets kept in a pill box and carried with the patient deteriorate in a week.

Advises Dr. Mayer: Buy a supply of one hundred tablets. They should be in the original factory bottle of amber glass with metal screw cap—not dispensed in a pharmacy plastic container. Write the purchase date on the bottle, remove the cotton stuffer, and keep the bottle tightly capped in the refrigerator. Once a week, open the bottle to remove as many tablets as are likely to be needed for the next week. Carry these with you in any type of container and, after a week, discard any that remain unused.   (D-15)

References

ALLERGIES

A-1.   *Journal of Allergy and Clinical Immunology*, 56:222.

A-2.   *Medical Tribune*, August 6, 1975, p. 19.

A-3.   *Annals of Allergy*, 29:356.

A-4.   *Annals of Allergy*, 28:87.

A-5.   *Archives of Dermatology*, 108:537.

A-6.   *Archives of Dermatology*, 110:921.

A-7.   Report to American Academy of Dermatology by Dr. William F. Schorr, Marshfield Clinic, Marshfield, Wis.

A-8.   Report from the American Medical Association based on work by Drs. W. P. Jordan, Jr., and M. C. Bourlas, Medical College of Virginia, Richmond.

A-9.   Drs. Jacob Brem and Malm Weeratne, Worcester (Mass.) City Hospital.

A-10.   *Annals of Allergy*, 28:371.

A-11.   *Journal of Allergy and Clinical Immunology*, 53:200.

A-12.   Dr. Alan A. Wanderer, National Jewish Hospital and Research Center, Denver, Colo.

A-13.   *American Family Physician*, vol. 13, no. 2, p. 106.

ARTHRITIS AND MUSCULOSKELETAL DISORDERS

AM-1.   *Journal of the American Medical Association*, 233:336; 233:364.

AM-2.   *American Family Physician*, vol. 13, no. 2, p. 116.

AM-3.   Report to American Society of Anesthesiologists by Dr. Harold Carron, University of Virginia Medical School, Charlottesville.

AM-4.   *Arthritis and Rheumatism*, 16:139.

AM-5.   Report to American Rheumatism Association by Dr. Robert Godfrey, University of Kansas School of Medicine.

AM-6.   *Arthroscope*, The Arthritis Foundation Newsletter, vol. 3, no. 2, Spring 1975.

AM-7.   *Archives of Physical Medicine and Rehabilitation*, 52:479.

AM-8.   *American Family Physician*, vol. 13, no. 2, p. 116.

AM-9.   Report to American Rheumatism Association by Drs. L. H. Milender and E. A. Nalebuff, Robert B. Brigham Hospital, Boston.

AM-10. *Clinical Orthopedics*, 95:9.

AM-11. *Clinical Orthopedics*, 94:171.

AM-12. *Medical World News*, vol. 15, no. 16, p. 40.

AM-13. *Medical Tribune*, October 8, 1975, p. 13.

AM-14. Report to American Rheumatism Association.

AM-15. Report from The Arthritis Foundation.

AM-16. *Journal of the American Medical Association*, 233:1247.

AM-17. *Journal of the American Medical Association*, 227:1373.

AM-18. Report from The Arthritis Foundation.

AM-19. *Medical Opinion*, vol. 4, no. 9, p. 35.

AM-20. *Journal of the American Medical Association*, 231:1143.

AM-21. *Canadian Medical Association Journal*, 111:137.

AM-22. *Archives of Neurology*, 17:503.

AM-23. *Medical World News*, vol. 14, no. 41, p. 86D.

AM-24. *The Medical Letter on Drugs & Therapeutics*, vol. 16, no. 15.

AM-25. Report to American Medical Association 119th convention.

AM-26. *Medical World News*, vol. 15, no. 9, p. 22.

CANCER

C-1. Report to American Cancer Society Seminar for Science Writers, 1976.

C-2. Report to Royal College of Physicians and Surgeons, Quebec City, 1976.

C-3. *New England Journal of Medicine*, 294:405.

C-4. *Journal of the American Medical Association*, 235:1049.

C-5. Report to Symposium on Combined Modality Therapy of Cancer, Denver.

C-6. *Canadian Medical Association Journal*, 112:308.

C-7. *Medical World News*, vol. 16, no. 4, p. 63.

EAR DISORDERS

EA-1. *Archives of Neurology*, 27:129.

EA-2. *Archives of Otolaryngology*, 100:262.

EA-3. *Medical Tribune*, vol. 15, no. 2, p. 21.

EA-4. *Medical World News*, vol. 12, no. 39, p. 34E.

EA-5. *The Laryngoscope*, 5:639.

EA-6.   *Archives of Otolaryngology*, 97:118.

EA-7.   *Medical World News*, vol. 15, no. 27, p. 44H; vol. 16, no. 4, p. 47.

EA-8.   Report from the American Academy of Pediatrics.

EA-9.   *Archives of Otolaryngology*, 93:183.

EA-10.   Report from American Academy of Ophthalmology and Otolaryngology.

EA-11.   Report from the American Academy of Family Physicians.

EA-12.   Report from the American Medical Association.

EA-13.   *Journal of the American Medical Association*, 227:1165.

EA-14.   *Archives of Otolaryngology*, 98:10.

EMOTIONAL/BEHAVIORAL PROBLEMS

EB-1.   *Science News*, 108:277.

EB-2.   Kline, N. S., *From Sad to Glad*, Putnam, N.Y., 1974.

EB-3.   *American Family Physician*, 102:99.
Journal of the American Medical Association, 227:1158.
Learning About Depressive Illness, National Institute of Mental Health, DHEW Publication (HSM) 72-9110.
Galton, L., *Don't Give Up on an Aging Parent*, Crown, 1975.
Solomon, K., "On Dementia and Pseudodementia," *Medical World News*, vol. 15, no. 38, p. 16.
British Journal of Psychiatry, 119:39.

EB-4.   *American Journal of Psychiatry*, 126:1667.

EB-5.   *Medical Tribune*, vol. 15, no. 36, p. 1.

EB-6.   *American Family Physician*, vol. 10, no. 4, p. 196.
American Journal of Psychiatry, 131: 198.
Lithium: Its Role in Psychiatric Research and Treatment, ed. by S. Gerson and B. Shopsin, Plenum.

EB-7.   *Archives of General Psychiatry*, 27:519.

EB-8.   *British Medical Journal*, 4(1974):633.

EB-9.   *American Journal of Psychology*, 131:1089.

EYE DISORDERS

E-1.   *Medical Journal of Australia*, 2(1973):337.

E-2.   *Journal of the American Medical Association*, 219:93.

E-3.   *Journal of the American Medical Association*, 227:79.

E-4.   Scientific exhibit, American Association of Ophthalmologists and Otolaryngologists, Dallas meeting.

E-5.   Report to American Academy of Ophthalmology and Otolaryngology.

E-6.   Report to American Academy of Ophthalmology and Otolaryngology.

E-7.   *Medical World News*, vol. 15, no. 9, p. 13.

E-8.   *Annals of Otology, Rhinology and Laryngology*, 81:611.

E-9.   Symposium, New Orleans Academy of Ophthalmology.

E-10.   Report to Research to Prevent Blindness Seminar.

GASTROINTESTINAL DISORDERS

GI-1.   *Annals of Internal Medicine*, 80:573.

GI-2.   *British Medical Journal*, 3(1972):793.

GI-3.   *Journal of the American Medical Association*, 225:1243.

GI-4.   Galton, L., *The Truth About Fiber in Your Diet*, Crown, 1976.

GI-5.   *Gastroenterology*, 63:399.

GI-6.   Report to American College of Gastroenterology.

GI-7.   Report from the American Medical Association.

GI-8.   *Journal of the American Medical Association*, 226:1525.

GI-9.   *Journal of the American Medical Association*, 217:1359.

GI-10.   Galton, L., *The Truth About Fiber in Your Diet*, Crown, 1976.

GI-11.   *Medical World News*, vol. 15, no. 13, p. 22.

GI-12.   *Archives of Otolaryngology*, 92:499.

GI-13.   *Journal of the American Medical Association*, 225:1659.

GI-14.   Report to American Dietetic Association.

GI-15.   Report to Cleveiand General Hospital Symposium.

GI-16.   Report from the American Medical Association.

GENITOURINARY DISORDERS

GU-1.   *New York State Journal of Medicine*, 71:2865.

GU-2.   *Medical World News*, vol. 15, no. 36, p. 16.

GU-3.   Report from Michael Reese Medical Center, Chicago.

GU-4.   *Journal of the National Cancer Institute*, 53:335.

GU-5.   Report to the American Medical Association.

GU-6.   Reports to American Urological Association.
         Medical World News, vol. 15, no. 24, p. 17.

GU-7.   *Medical Tribune*, vol. 14, no. 46, p. 1.

GU-8.   Report from the American Medical Association.

GU-9.   *Hospital Practice*, vol. 9, no. 11, p. 143.

GU-10. *Dialysis and Transplantation*, June-July, 1975.
Surgery, 75:447.
Surgery, Gynecology and Obstetrics, 141:69.
American Journal of Surgery, 128:54.
Archives of Surgery, 110:114.

GU-11. *Journal of the American Medical Association*, 233:787.

GU-12. Report from American College of Surgeons.

GERIATRIC PROBLEMS

GE-1.   Galton, L., *Don't Give Up on an Aging Parent*, Crown, 1975.

GE-2.   *Radiology*, 116:85.

GE-3.   *Journal of the American Geriatric Society*, 20:127.

GE-4.   *Medical World News*, vol. 16, no. 24, p. 52.

GE-5.   *American Family Physician*, vol. 10, no. 6, p. 91.

GE-6.   *Journal of the American Medical Association*, 217:1036.

GE-7.   *American Family Physician*, vol. 10, no. 1, p. 111.

GE-8.   *American Family Physician*, vol. 8, no. 4, p. 243.

GE-9.   *American Family Physician*, vol. 8, no. 3, p. 213.

GE-10. *Journal of the American Medical Association*, 234:960.

GE-11. *Medical Tribune*, vol. 14, no. 34, p. 8.

GE-12. Report from American Society of Abdominal Surgeons.

GE-13. *Archives of Surgery*, 110:1107.

GE-14. *Annals of Thoracic Surgery*, 18:81.

GE-15. *Archives of Surgery*, 107:30.

HEADACHES

H-1.   Report to American College of Allergists.

H-2.   *Canadian Medical Association Journal*, 109:891.

H-3.   *American Family Physician*, vol. 6, no. 6, p. 60.

H-4.   *Modern Medicine*, vol. 40, no. 20, p. 128.

H-5.   *Headache*, 15:36.

H-6.   *Neurology*, 22:366.

H-7.   *Medical World News*, vol. 12, no. 14, p. 13.
Reports from Menninger Foundation, Topeka, Kansas, and
Long Island Jewish Hospital-Hillside Medical Center, New
Hyde Park, N.Y.

H-8.   *Archives of Neurology,* 32:649.

H-9.   *Today's Health,* March 1973, p. 7.

H-10.   *Journal of the American Medical Association,* 221:1165.

H-11.   *American Family Physician,* vol. 11, no. 5, p. 105.
        American Journal of Diseases of Childhood, 120:122.

HEART DISEASE

HT-1.   *American Heart Journal,* 87:722.

HT-2.   *American Journal of Medicine,* 55:583.

HT-3.   *Lancet,* 1(1973):1404.

HT-4.   Report to American Association of Pathologists and Bacteriologists.

HT-5.   Report to American College of Physicians.

HT-6.   Report to American Heart Association.

HT-7.   *Lancet,* 1(1973):333.

HT-8.   *Journal of the American Medical Association,* 230:130.

HT-9.   Galton, L., *The Silent Disease: Hypertension,* Crown, 1973.

HT-10. *The Good Drugs Do,* Special Supplement, Medical Tribune.

HT-11. *Journal of Human Stress,* 2:24.

HT-12. Gentry, W. D., and Williams, R. B., Jr., *Psychological Aspects of Myocardial Infarction and Coronary Care,* Mosby, 1975.

HT-13. Report from Tufts-New England Medical Center.

HT-14. *American Journal of Cardiology,* 34:152.

HT-15. Reports to American Heart Association Symposium, Tucson.

HT-16. Likoff, W., et al., *Your Heart: Complete Information for the Family,* Lippincott, 1972.
        Castenada, A. R., et al., Reports to American Heart Association Forum for Science Writers, Marco Island, Fla.

NEUROLOGIC DISORDERS

N-1.   *Journal of the American Medical Association,* 227:327.

N-2.   Report to American Academy for Cerebral Palsy, Dr. Eric Denhoff, Meeting Street School Children's Rehabilitation Center, Providence, R.I.

N-3.   *Journal of the American Medical Association,* 229:1755.

N-4.   Report to American Academy of Neurology, Dr. N. T. Mathew, Baylor College of Medicine, Houston.

N-5.   *Journal of the American Medical Association*, 229:552.

N-6.   *Neurology*, 25:515.

N-7.   *Medical World News*, vol. 15, no. 38, p. 9.

N-8.   *Archives of Neurology*, 198:204.

N-9.   *Journal of the American Medical Association*, 233:278.

N-10.   *Medical World News*, vol. 15, no. 23, p. 30K.

N-11.   Report to First International Congress of Child Neurology, To-
        ronto.

N-12.   Report to American Pediatric Society.

N-13.   Report to American Epilepsy Society.

N-14.   *Journal of the American Medical Association*, 233:535.

N-15.   *Medical World News*, vol. 15, no. 39, p. 59.

N-16.   Report to American Academy of Neurology.

N-17.   *Neurology*, 24:795.

N-18.   *American Journal of Surgery*, 128:202.

N-19.   *American Journal of Medicine*, 50:465.

N-20.   Report from Michael Reese Medical Center, Chicago.

N-21.   *New York State Journal of Medicine*, 73:2657.

N-22.   *Journal of Neurosurgery*, 39:235.

N-23.   *Medical Tribune*, "In Consultation," December 17, 1975, p. 6.

N-24.   Report to American Heart Association.

N-25.   *Stroke*, 5:76.

N-26.   *Lancet*, 1(1973):1407.

N-27.   Report to American Heart Association.

OBSTETRICS AND GYNECOLOGY

OB-1.   *New England Journal of Medicine*, 293:573.

OB-2.   *Obstetrics and Gynecology*, 35:937.

OB-3.   *Science News*, 108:267.

OB-4.   Report to North American Conference on Fertility and Sterility,
        Dr. H. W. Horne, Jr.

OB-5.   *Harefuah*, 89:201.

OB-6.   *Medical Tribune*, vol. 14, no. 9, p. 23.

OB-7.   *American Journal of Obstetrics and Gynecology*, 112:213.

OB-8.   *Canadian Medical Association Journal*, 109:1104.

OB-9.   *Lancet*, August 23, 1975.

OB-10. *American Journal of Obstetrics and Gynecology*, 112:1101.

OB-11.   Report to Sixth World Congress of Gynecology.

OB-12.   *Journal of the American Medical Association*, 226:1521.

OB-13.   *Obstetrics and Gynecology*, 44:637.

OB-14.   *Journal of Obstetrics and Gynecology British Commonwealth*, 80:718.

OB-15.   *New England Journal of Medicine*, 294:393.
          Hospital Practice, vol. 10, no. 6, p. 41.
          Maternal/Newborn Advocate (National Foundation), vol. 2, no. 4, p. 3.

OB-16.   *American Journal of Obstetrics and Gynecology*, 109:850.

OB-17.   *Medical World News*, vol. 14, no. 46, p. 80M.

OB-18.   *Medical World News*, vol. 13, no. 11, p. 44H.

OB-19.   *Medical World News*, vol. 16, no. 4, p. 111.

OB-20.   *Canadian Medical Association Journal*, 107:496.

OB-21.   Report to American College of Surgeons.
          Fertility and Sterility, 26:217.

OB-22.   Report to American College of Surgeons.

OB-23.   *Science News*, 104:182.

OB-24.   *Modern Medicine*, vol. 40, no. 19, p. 31.

OB-25.   *New York State Journal of Medicine*, 73:559.

OB-26.   Report to Federal Agency for International Development.

OB-27.   *Medical World News*, vol. 16, no. 12, p. 7.

OB-28.   *Journal of the American Medical Association*, 225:507.

OB-29.   *American Journal of Obstetrics and Gynecology*, 117:453.

OB-30.   Report to American Society of Clinical Pathologists.

OB-31.   *New York State Journal of Medicine*, 75:1443.

OB-32.   *Obstetrics and Gynecology*, 43:893.

OB-33.   Dr. M. C. Rulin, in *Family Practice*, ed. H. F. Conn et al., Saunders, 1973.

OB-34.   *Journal of the American Medical Association*, 231:934.

OB-35.   *Journal of the American Medical Association*, 229:641.

OB-36.   *Medical Tribune*, vol. 15, no. 9, p. 3.

OB-37.   *Obstetrics and Gynecology*, 43:797.

OB-38.   *Journal of the American Medical Association*, 221:304.

OB-39.   Report to American Urological Association.

PEDIATRICS

P-1.   Report from National Institute of Mental Health.

P-2.   *Child Development*, 42:399.

P-3.   *Medical World News*, vol. 15, no. 26, p. 13.

P-4.   Report from American Academy of Pediatrics.

P-5.   *American Journal of Diseases of Children*, 125:30.

P-6.   *American Journal of Diseases of Children*, 117:458.

P-7.   *American Family Physician*, vol. 7, no. 5, p. 180.

P-8.   Report from American Academy of Pediatrics.

P-9.   *Journal of the American Medical Association*, 212:2231.

P-10.   *American Journal of Diseases of Children*, 121:219.

P-11.   *Pediatrics*, 54:196.

P-12.   Report from American College of Radiology.

P-13.   *Pediatrics*, 50:429.

P-14.   *Journal of the American Medical Association*, 222:65.

P-15.   *Medical Tribune*, vol. 15, no. 6, p. 1.

P-16.   *American Family Physician*, vol. 9, no. 4, p. 191.

P-17.   Report to Society for Pediatric Research.

P-18.   *Medical Journal of Australia*, (1971):307.

P-19.   *Pediatric Review*, 6:868.

P-20.   *American Journal of Diseases of Children*, 129:1397.

P-21.   *Pediatrics*, 50:874.

P-22.   *American Journal of Diseases of Children*, 128:21.

P-23.   *Archives of Otolaryngology*, 101:591.

P-24.   *American Family Physician*, vol. 13, no. 3, p. 171.
        Report to Canadian Pediatric Society.

P-25.   *Journal of the American Medical Association*, 225:610.

P-26.   *Journal of Pediatrics*, 86:697.

P-27.   *Clinical Pediatrics*, 10:336.

P-28.   *Journal of the American Medical Association*, 225:1132.

P-29.   Report from American Academy of Pediatrics.

RESPIRATORY DISEASES

R-1.   *Pediatrics*, 48:939.

R-2.   *Medical World News*, May 13, 1972, p. 33.

R-3.   *American Family Physician*, vol. 11, no. 3, p. 74.

R-4.   Report to American Academy of Allergy by Dr. D. R. Miklich,
        National Asthma Center, Denver.

R-5.   *Archives of Otolaryngology*, 100:109.

R-6.   *Journal of Allergy and Clinical Immunology*, 49:348.

R-7.   Report to American Academy of Pediatrics.

R-8.   *Journal of the American Medical Association*, 227:1061.

R-9.   *Medical Journal of Australia*, (1974):158.

R-10.   *American Family Physician*, vol. 11, no. 3, p. 74.

R-11.   *Journal of the American Medical Association*, 233:804.

R-12.   *Journal of the American Medical Association*, 234:295.

R-13.   *Medical Tribune*, vol. 14, no. 35, p. 5.

R-14.   *Journal of Infectious Diseases*, January 1976.

R-15.   *New England Journal of Medicine*, 288:1361.

R-16.   *Journal of the American Medical Association*, 227:164.

R-17.   Stanford University Symposium on vitamin C.

R-18.   *Canadian Medical Association Journal*, 112:823.

R-19.   *Executive Health*, vol. 12, no. 3, Executive Publications, Pickfair Bldg., Rancho Santa Fe, Calif. 92067.

R-20.   *American Family Physician*, vol. 10, no. 5, p. 215.

R-21.   Report to American Academy of Pediatrics by Dr. J. C. Adair.

R-22.   Report from American Medical Association.

SKIN, HAIR, AND NAILS

S-1.   *Archives of Dermatology*, February 1973.

S-2.   *Archives of Dermatology*, 106:200.

S-3.   *Medical World News*, vol. 15, no. 34, p. 15 and vol. 15, no. 42, p. 56.

S-4.   *Medical Tribune*, vol. 14, no. 29, p. 9.

S-5.   *American Family Physician*, vol. 3, no. 3, p. 102.

S-6.   *Journal of the American Medical Association*, 224:257.

S-7.   *Medical Tribune*, January 10, 1973.

S-8.   Report to American Medical Association.

S-9.   *Journal of the American Medical Association*, 229:60.

S-10.   *Archives of Dermatology*, 111:1004.

S-11.   *Journal of American Podiatry Association*, 61:382.

S-12.   *Journal of the American Medical Association*, 224:905.

S-13.   *Medical World News*, vol. 15, no. 42, p. 15.

S-14.   *Medical Tribune*, vol. 14, no. 9, p. 11.

S-15.   *Medical World News*, vol. 15, no. 38, p. 39.

S-16. *Journal of the American Medical Association,* 228:157.

S-17. *Journal of the American Medical Association,* 219:519.

S-18. *Medical World News,* vol. 15, no. 28, p. 51.

S-19. Report to Medical Society of the State of New York, by Dr. Robert Auerbach.

S-20. Report from the American Medical Association.

S-21. *Journal of the American Medical Association,* 231:1026.

S-22. *Journal of the American Medical Association,* 233:1257.

S-23. *Cutis,* 9:375.

S-24. *Medical World News,* vol. 13, no. 39, p. 84.

S-25. *Journal of the American Medical Association,* 230:878.

S-26. *Medical World News,* vol. 14, no. 40, p. 14K.

S-27. *Journal of the American Medical Association,* 224:132.

S-28. *Journal of the American Medical Association,* 210:2341.

S-29. Report from the American Medical Association.

S-30. *Medical World News,* vol. 17, no. 1, p. 89.

S-31. *Journal of the American Medical Association,* 228:1004.

S-32. *American Family Physician,* vol. 9, no. 6, p. 70.

S-33. *Journal of the American Medical Association,* 230:72.

S-34. *Science News,* 103:240.

S-35. *Archives of Dermatology,* 107:580.

S-36. *American Family Physician,* vol. 9, no. 6, p. 70.

SLEEP

SL-1. *Archives of General Psychiatry,* 26:463.

SL-2. *Fortune,* June 1975, p. 158.

SL-3. *Medical World News,* vol. 12, no. 5, p. 286.

SL-4. *Modern Medicine,* vol. 40, no. 17, p. 40.

SL-5. *Journal of the American Medical Association,* 227:514.

SL-6. Report to American Psychological Association.

SL-7. *Journal of the American Medical Association,* 230:1680.

SL-8. *Science News,* October 4, 1975.

SL-9. *Journal of the American Medical Association,* 220:1745.

SL-10. *Journal of the American Medical Association,* 219:394.

SL-11. *Journal of the American Medical Association,* 228:978.

OTHER PROBLEMS, OTHER DEVELOPMENTS

OP-1. *Journal of the American Medical Association*, 225:1532.

OP-2. *American Family Physician*, vol. 12, no. 5, p. 131.

OP-3. *American Family Physician*, vol. 11, no. 4, p. 93.

OP-4. *Journal of the American Medical Association*, 233:42.

OP-5. Report from the University of Chicago.

OP-6. *New England Journal of Medicine*, 293:893.

OP-7. Report to American Dental Association.

OP-8. Report to International Association for Dental Research.

OP-9. *American Family Practice*, vol. 6, no. 5, p. 77.
Report to American Dental Association by Dr. B. W. Kwapis, Southern Illinois University School of Dental Medicine.

OP-10. Report to International Association for Dental Research.

OP-11. Report to Federation of American Societies for Experimental Biology.

OP-12. Report to American Diabetes Association.

OP-13. Report from National Institutes of Health by Dr. Carl Kupfer, Director of National Eye Institute.

OP-14. Report to Gastroenterology Research Group by Dr. Stephen Goldfinger, Massachusetts General Hospital, Boston.

OP-15. *Medical Opinion and Review*, vol. 6, no. 5.

OP-16. *Medical World News*, vol. 16, no. 27, p. 9.

OP-17. *Southern Medical Journal*, 67:1308.
California Medicine, 111:87.

OP-18. *Journal of the American Medical Association*, 230:374.

OP-19. *Journal of the American Medical Association*, 223:627.
Report by Dr. Ralph A. Nelson to Federation of American Societies for Experimental Biology.

OP-20. *Archives of Physical Medicine and Rehabilitation*, 53:323.

OP-21. Report from American Medical Association.

OP-22. *Annals of Internal Medicine*, 127:408.

OP-23. *New York State Journal of Medicine*, 74:1563.

OP-24. *Psychosomatic Medicine*, 33:49.

OP-25. Report to American Medical Association, by Dr. A. J. Stunkard.

OP-26. Report to American Academy of Orthopedic Surgeons.

OP-27. *American Family Physician*, vol. 8, no. 6, p. 75.

OP-28. Report to American Federation for Clinical Research.

OP-29. *Chest*, 68:195.

OP-30.   *American Family Physician*, vol. 13, no. 1, p. 78.

OP-31.   *Archives of Dermatology*, 110:233.

OP-32.   *Journal of the American Medical Association*, 225:739.

OP-33.   *Journal of the American Medical Association*, 223:801.

OP-34.   Report to American Academy of Orthopedic Surgeons.

OP-35.   Report to American Thyroid Association.

OP-36.   Report to American College of Chest Surgeons.

OP-37.   *Journal of the American Medical Association*, 226:1247.

OP-38.   Report from the American Medical Association.

OP-39.   *Behavioral Research and Therapy*, 12:279.

OP-40.   *Medical World News*, vol. 13, no. 37, p. 68; Report to American Academy of Orthopedic Surgeons.

OP-41.   Report to American Academy of Orthopedic Surgeons.

OP-42.   *Western Journal of Medicine*, 122:450.

DRUGS AND DRUG TAKING

D-1.   Report from University of Rochester.

D-2.   *Hospital Practice*, January 1976.

D-3.   *Canadian Medical Association Journal*, 110:1346.

D-4.   Miller, B. F., and Galton, L., *The Family Book of Preventive Medicine*, Simon & Schuster.

D-5.   *American Journal of Nursing*, 75:402.

D-6.   Report to American Gastroenterological Association.

D-7.   *British Medical Journal*, (1975):21.

D-8.   Report to American College of Surgeons by Dr. René Menguy, University of Chicago.

D-9.   *Journal of the American Medical Association*, 230:1385.

D-10.   *American Dental Association News*, vol. 6, no. 12, p. 6.

D-11.   Report from the American Dental Association.

D-12.   *Journal of the American Medical Association*, 216:1352.

D-13.   Report to American Heart Association.

D-14.   *Journal of the American Medical Association*, 219:176.

D-15.   *Canadian Medical Association Journal*, 110:788.

Index